KHYBER PAKHTUNKHWA
HEALTH SECTOR REVIEW

HOSPITAL CARE

OCTOBER 2019

ADB

ASIAN DEVELOPMENT BANK

© 2019 Asian Development Bank
6 ADB Avenue, Mandaluyong City, 1550 Metro Manila, Philippines
Tel +63 2 8632 4444; Fax +63 2 8636 2444
www.adb.org

Some rights reserved. Published in 2019.

ISBN 978-92-9261-764-6 (print), 978-92-9261-765-3 (electronic)
Publication Stock No. TCS190481-2
DOI: http://dx.doi.org/10.22617/TCS190481-2

Notes:
In this publication, "$" refers to United States dollars.

On the cover: Hospital bed and overcrowded patients in Khyber Pakhtunkhwa (photos by Mr. Hiddo Huitzing and Michael Niechzial).
Cover design by Francis Manio.

CONTENTS

Tables, Figures, and Boxes   v

Foreword   vii

Preface   viii

Acknowledgments   ix

Abbreviations   x

CHAPTER 1
Introduction   1
   I   Overview   1
   II Provincial Socioeconomic and Health Sector Context   1
   III Purpose and Scope   4
   IV Methodology   5

CHAPTER 2
Health Governance   6
   I   Overview   6
   II Achievements   6
   III Challenges   8
   IV Recommendations   16

CHAPTER 3
Health Infrastructure   18
   I   Overview   18
   II Achievements   18
   III Current Status   19
   IV Challenges   24
   V   Recommendations   33

CHAPTER 4
Health Financing — 37

I   Overview — 37

II   Achievements — 37

III Current Status and Challenges — 38

IV   Recommendations — 46

References — 48

Appendixes — 51

1 Case Study on Hospital Contracting Experience in Khyber Pakhtunkhwa — 51
2 Key Elements of a Strong Contract — 56
3 Methodology for Modeling Demand for Health Care — 57
4 Continuous Quality Improvement Description and Good Practice Examples of Standard Operating Procedures for Medical Care — 58
5 Financing Sources by Financing Agents, FY2016 — 64
6 Overview of Population Segments Receiving Financial Coverage for Health — 66
7 Social Health Protection Initiative: Sehat Sahulat Program — 70
8 Actuarial Projections of Supply and Demand-Side Interventions in the Khyber Pakhtunkhwa Health Sector — 73

TABLES, FIGURES, AND BOXES

Tables

1	Health Facility Network	11
2	Authority Lines and Responsibilities for Health Facilities	12
3	Distribution of Selected Payment Responsibilities across Public Facilities	13
4	Inpatient Admission per 1,000 Population, 2009–2015	24
5	Outpatient Visits per Capita, 2009–2015	24
6	Performance Data of the Most Frequented Secondary Level Hospitals, 2017	28
7	Inpatient Services at Surveyed Hospitals	30
8	Projected Demand for Episodes and Capacity for Dialysis, 2020–2035	30
9	Planned and Filled Health Workforce, 2018	31
10	Health Workforce Composition at Surveyed Hospitals	32
11	Consolidated Current Budget of Health Sector	40
12	Consolidated Allocations by Major Line Items	42
13	Current Health Expenditures by Activities, 2015–2016	43
14	Consolidated Current Budget and Expenditure of Secondary Care Facilities	44
A1	Status of Facility Boards	55
A2	Overview of Phases of the Social Health Protection Initiative (Sehat Sahulat Program)	72

Figures

1	World Health Organization´s Dimensions of Health Sector Governance	8
2	Public Health Facilities by Hierarchy of Service Provision	20
3	Health Care System and Service Delivery	21
4	Proportion of Doctors in the Public Sector and Population by Districts, 2017	22
5	Proportion of Nurses in the Public Sector and Population by Districts, 2017	23

6   Good Example of Quality Improvement Tools and Mechanisms   35
     (Guidelines/Clinical Pathways) for Patients with Symptoms of Heart Failure

7   Flow of Government Funds to Health Facilities   39

8   Sectoral Share of Health Budget Allocations: Trend Analysis   40

9   National Health Accounts, 2015–2016   41

10   Average Allocation (5 Years) by Items of Expenditure for Secondary Care Hospitals   44

11   Expenditure Mix—Salary and Non-Salary (Secondary Health Care Facilities)   45

A1   Elements of a Strong Contract   56

Boxes

     Standards for Intensive Care Unit Adjacencies: Health Building Notes   26
     of the United Kingdom's National Health Service

A1   World Health Organization Health Systems Framework   62
     and Quality of Care

FOREWORD

The Asian Development Bank (ADB) has been providing technical and financial support to the health sector in Pakistan, particularly the Khyber Pakhtunkhwa Province, for the last 2 decades. ADB's Operational Plan for Health 2015–2020 identifies three key areas of investment for supporting the developing member countries achieve universal health coverage.

Knowing that good governance guided by a health systems approach promotes effective delivery of health services and that investment in health care leads to economic growth, the Government of Khyber Pakhtunkhwa desires to lead the province in the 21st century with approaches that are in tandem with international best practices, taking guidance from global research and local circumstances. The main strategies for taking forward this intent would be (i) strengthening health systems for better governance; and (ii) collaborating with health and non-health sectors, public and private sectors, and the citizens for a shared vision and interest. Further, delivering quality health care services to all is the goal of the Government of Khyber Pakhtunkhwa, which seeks to improve the health status of an increasing number of citizens on an equal basis through expanded access to effective essential health care, backed by adequate referral services and resources.

Health is coexistent with other sectors such as economy, environment, education, transport, food security, and other non-health sectors. A holistic approach is necessary to achieve the desired objectives of a better performing health sector.

What makes this assessment unique is the focus on hospital care, which the previous assessments disregarded. The insights into health governance, hospital autonomy, contracting, infrastructure, status of physical and human resources, projections on demand for inpatient services, quality of hospital care, and health financing have brought up a key recommendation that the Department of Health will closely review and try to incorporate in its updated health sector strategic directions.

I would like to offer my gratitude to ADB for commissioning this health sector review, bringing a cross-national team of experts, and organizing the events leading to this conclusion.

Farooq Jamil
Secretary Health, Government of Khyber Pakhtunkhwa

PREFACE

As a founding member of the Asian Development Bank (ADB), Pakistan has a long history of collaboration with ADB. Together, much progress has been made in accelerating the country's economic and social advancement and addressing developmental needs across multiple sectors.

Pakistan has typically experienced more challenges in improving health outcomes than other countries in South and East Asia. Health is a critical contributor to a country's economic and social prosperity, and therefore it is vital for governments to prioritize this sector when considering development objectives. With relatively high infant mortality, neonatal mortality, and maternal mortality, Pakistan has long way to go to meet the Sustainable Development Goals on health.

Located in the northwestern region of Pakistan, Khyber Pakhtunkhwa is the smallest province geographically, characterized by high population growth and a large refugee population. It faces a set of unique obstacles in the health sector including poor access and utilization of services, low financial protection, and weak governance.

This report was commissioned at the request of the government to identify bottlenecks and opportunities within the focus areas of health governance, health infrastructure, and health financing in the framework of hospital care. It is only a starting point for creating a comprehensive health strategy that will guide the government, development partners, and policy makers as they prioritize investments and projects in the health sector.

Since 1966, ADB has supported Pakistan in strengthening the country's key infrastructure and social services while promoting economic growth. Our hope is to build on this historic partnership with the newly elected government, to one day provide universal health coverage in Khyber Pakhtunkhwa and in Pakistan.

Werner Liepach
Director General
Central and West Asia Department

ACKNOWLEDGMENTS

This review was prepared by a team led by Rouselle F. Lavado, senior health specialist, and Faraz Khalid, consultant, of the Social Sector Division (CWSS) of the Central and West Asia Department of the Asian Development Bank (ADB). Team members Munir Abro, Eduardo Banzon, Andrea Godon, and Hiddo Huitzing (ADB); and consultants Jamal Afridi, Ammar Aftab, Bernard Couttolenc, Nasir Idrees, Zahra Ladhani, Martina Merten, Frances Ng, and Michael Niechzial contributed to the review. Khyber Medical University conducted the survey of medical facilities.

Peer reviewers Fahad Hasan and Ayesha Jamshaid provided valuable comments.

Rose Anne G. Dumayas provided meticulous quality control and managed the production of the report. Madeline Dizon, Wendy Montealto, and Jenalyn Soubiron provided administrative support.

The team is grateful for the support from the following: Rie Hiraoka, director, CWSS; Patrick Osewe, chief, Health Sector Group, Sustainable Development and Climate Change Department; and Xiaohong Yang, country director, Pakistan Resident Mission.

SherGul of the Ministry of Health represented the government team in coordinating the review. The team appreciates the close collaboration of the Government of Khyber Paktunkhwa, the Ministry of Health and the Sehat Sahulat Program, and the Ministry of Finance. Key informants and workshop participants also provided useful comments to the background papers.

Development partners—the Department for International Development of the United Kingdom, the GiZ, the Japan International Cooperation Agency, the KfW, the United States Agency for International Development, the World Health Organization, and the World Bank—provided valuable inputs.

ABBREVIATIONS

A&E	accident and emergency
ADB	Asian Development Bank
ALOS	average length of stay
BHU	basic health unit
CQI	continuous quality improvement
DHIS	district health information system
DHO	district health officer
DHQ	district headquarter
DOH	Department of Health
ENT	ear, nose, throat
EPR	electronic patient record
GDP	gross domestic product
HCC	Health Care Commission
HMIS	health management information system
HRH	human resources for health
HSS	Health Sector Strategy
ICU	intensive care unit
IMU	independent monitoring unit
KMU	Khyber Medical University
M&E	monitoring and evaluation
MHSDP	minimum health services delivery package
MTI	medical teaching institution
NGO	nongovernment organization
NHSRC	National Health Services, Regulations and Coordination
OOP	out-of-pocket

OPD	outpatient department
PFM	public financial management
PHC	primary health care
PMT	proxy means testing
PPHI	People's Primary Healthcare Initiative
PPP	public–private partnership
RHC	rural health center
SHPI	social health protection initiative
SLIC	State Life Insurance Corporation of Pakistan
SOP	standard operating procedure
THQ	*tehsil* headquarters
UHC	universal health coverage
WHO	World Health Organization

CHAPTER 1

Introduction

I.   Overview

In 2017, the Department of Health (DOH) of the Government of Khyber Pakhtunkhwa requested the Asian Development Bank (ADB) to commission a health sector review focusing on health governance, health infrastructure, and the health financing aspects of hospital care. The key objectives of the review were to identify bottlenecks and opportunities within the three focus areas and to lay the foundation for the development of a sector-wide Khyber Pakhtunkhwa health plan. The review was based on a critical appraisal of current documents and data available in the DOH and allied offices, a quantitative survey of 30 secondary care hospitals, and two missions to Khyber Pakhtunkhwa in November 2017 and February 2018. This section broadly outlines the socioeconomic profile of the province and the health sector context, as well as the scope, purpose, and methodology of the review.

II.   Provincial Socioeconomic and Health Sector Context

Socioeconomic Status

Khyber Pakhtunkhwa is in the northwestern region of Pakistan and is one of the country's four administrative provinces. Although Khyber Pakhtunkhwa is the smallest province geographically with 7 divisions and 26 districts,[1] its total population has increased from 17.7 million in 1998 to 30.5 million in 2017 according to recent census estimates, and the population growth rate (2.89%) exceeds the national rate (2.40%). The vast majority of the population reside in rural areas (81%), with a few densely populated urban centers including Peshawar, which has a population of 2.1 million.[2] Over 3 million Afghan refugees are estimated to be residing in the province.

Following several years of conflict and political instability, the province currently faces considerable challenges that have restricted economic and social progress. The economic activity in the province has been negatively impacted due to an influx of refugees, violence, and a prolonged state of insecurity. With an underdeveloped manufacturing sector, the main sources of economic activity come from the forestry and agriculture sectors. The province generates 8% of Pakistan's

---

[1]   Due to a recent bill passed by the National Assembly of Pakistan, the Federally Administered Tribal Areas is set to be merged with Khyber Pakhtunkhwa. However, the administrative arrangements of this merger are still to be finalized.

[2]   Preliminary results from the 2017 census.

gross domestic product (GDP) with a per capita value of $800, half the national average per capita value.[3] The overall literacy rate is 54.1%, the lowest among the provinces; the literacy rate for females stands at an abysmal 36.8%.[4]

All urban households and 91.4% of rural households have access to electricity. More than 92% of the population (70% urban and 87% rural) own the house they reside in, while 92.7% of the population own a mobile phone. Solid fuel consumption for cooking is at a staggering 68%, which implies a high level of indoor pollution. However, 97% of these households do not cook in the room they sleep in. This measure is important for gauging physical proximity to indoor pollutants. It is also pertinent to note that of the 68% that use solid fuel for cooking, most are in rural areas. A majority of urban households (68%) use natural gas for cooking.[5]

Improved water and sanitation are accessible to 96.5% of urban and 86.5% of rural areas.[6] However, only 24.5% of the urban and 21.4% of the rural population use piped water. About 96% of urban and 81% of rural households have access to improved sanitation.[7] Overall, more than 77% of the population have access to both improved drinking water and sanitation; of this, 93% belong to urban and 72% to rural households (footnote 5).

Health Status

Pakistan has traditionally had poor health outcomes relative to other countries in South Asia and East Asia. In Khyber Pakhtunkhwa, many weaknesses and challenges have been identified in the current Health Sector Strategy (HSS),[8] including poor access to and utilization of health services, low quality and effectiveness of care, limited managerial capacity and weak accountability at all levels, systematic underfunding of the public health system, inefficient and inequitable resource allocation, low financial protection, and fragmented and discontinued reform initiatives.

The health outcomes of the province need substantial improvement and present an uphill task in achieving the Sustainable Development Goals. As per the Khyber Pakhtunkhwa Health Survey 2017, 67.5% of births were delivered in health facilities, but only 26.8% stayed for at least 12 hours for postnatal care (footnote 5). The neonatal mortality rate is 41 per 1,000 live births, the infant mortality rate is 58 per 1,000 live births, and the maternal mortality ratio is 206 per 100,000 live births.[9] Of children aged 12–23 months, 55.5% are reported to be fully immunized (based on records and mother's recall) (footnote 5). Approximately 17.3% of children aged 0–23 months have not received any vaccination at all. Over 40% of women have nutritional health problems

---

[3] Government of Khyber Pakhtunkhwa, Department of Finance.

[4] Government of Pakistan. *Labour Force Survey 2015.* http://www.pbs.gov.pk/sites/default/files/Annual%20Report%20 of%20LFS%202014-15.pdf.

[5] Khyber Pakhtunkhwa Health Survey 2017.

[6] According to the World Health Organization (WHO), "the category improved drinking water sources includes sources that, by nature of their construction or through active intervention, are protected from outside contamination, particularly faecal matter. These include piped water in a dwelling, plot or yard, and other improved sources." WHO. Drinking Water. https://www.who.int/water_sanitation_health/monitoring/water.pdf.

[7] According to WHO, an improved sanitation facility is defined as one that hygienically separates human excreta from human contact. WHO. Water Sanitation Hygiene. Key Terms. https://www.who.int/water_sanitation_health/monitoring/ jmp2012/key_terms/en/.

[8] Government of Khyber Pakhtunkhwa, DOH. 2010. *Khyber Pakhtunkhwa Health Sector Strategy 2010-2017.*

[9] Pakistan Social and Living Standards Measurement 2014-15; Population Census 2017; District Health Information System (DHIS) Khyber Pakhtunkhwa; Pakistan Demographic and Health Survey 2012-3; Interagency working group on maternal mortality ration in Pakistan; and Maternal, Newborn and Child Health Program.

(underweight, overweight or obese, anemic, iodine or zinc deficient), while 24% of children below 5 years of age are underweight, 48% are stunted, and 17% are wasted.[10]

Key Health Reforms

Several reforms have taken place in the health sector within the past decade. In 2010, the 18th Constitutional Amendment of Pakistan devolved health administration to the provinces, granting legislative as well executive authorities in the health sector, previously within the purview of the federal government, to the provinces.[11] At the time of devolution, Khyber Pakhtunkhwa already had the HSS 2010–2017 in place, but the process triggered a series of reforms aimed at addressing the unique challenges faced by the province with regard to strengthening the health system at large.

A key aspect of the devolution process has been electing local governments. The local government in Khyber Pakhtunkhwa has three tiers: district, *tehsil*,[12] and village. The mother and child health centers, rural health centers (RHCs), basic health units (BHUs), social welfare, population welfare, public health engineering, and public health hospitals have been devolved to the districts. Tertiary and teaching hospitals are devolved to the province. The devolution of financial power that allows the local governments to reallocate their assigned budget to areas of their choosing is among the most critical devolutions of powers to the local government and allows the local governments to deal with endemic and emergent issues within their jurisdiction more flexibly and effectively. The provincial government has been on an ambitious mission to reform the health landscape through various legal and programmatic initiatives.

Health policy in Khyber Pakhtunkhwa is informed mostly by the **Khyber Pakhtunkhwa HSS 2010–2017** and **National Health Vision 2016–2025**.[13] The provincial HSS 2010–2017 was extended until June 2018. Efforts are underway to update the strategy and align operational planning, midterm budgetary framework, and district-level health plans with this strategy.[14] Furthermore, since 2011, more than 23 ordinances/acts and amendments about health care have been passed in Khyber Pakhtunkhwa. Some of these are novel and introduce new dimensions in terms of quality, access, and service delivery, while others, mostly amendments, seek to update the existing laws. The most critical of these laws include (i) **Khyber Pakhtunkhwa Health Care Commission (HCC) Act, 2015**, which aims to regulate the health care in the province through sound technical knowledge; (ii) the **Khyber Pakhtunkhwa Public Health (Surveillance and Response) Ordinance, 2017**, the goal of which is to implement measures that help prevent and control diseases in the province; and (iii) the **Khyber Pakhtunkhwa Medical Teaching**

---

[10] Government of Pakistan, Ministry of National Health Services, Regulations and Coordination (NHSRC). 2012. *National Nutrition Survey 2011*. Islamabad.

[11] Constitution of the Islamic Republic of Pakistan, amend. 18, sec. 1.

[12] *Tehsil* is the second-lowest tier of local government in Pakistan. Each *tehsil* is subdivided into a number of union councils and is part of a larger district.

[13] The DOH, in collaboration with the Department for International Development of the United Kingdom (DFID), has recently started work on the new strategy. Due to the devolution of health to provincial governments in 2011, the national guiding health strategy—the National Health Vision—is no longer binding but has been serving as a guideline for provincial health policy. The National Health Vision identified eight thematic pillars for strengthening health systems in the country: sector governance, health financing, health service delivery, human resources for health, health information system and research, essential medicines and technology, cross-sectoral linkages, and global health responsibilities.

[14] The HSS defines five outcomes to be achieved in alignment with the provincial Comprehensive Development Strategy: Outcome 1: Enhanced coverage of and access to essential health services, especially for the poor and vulnerable; Outcome 2: Reduced morbidity and morbidity due to common diseases especially among vulnerable segments of the population; Outcome 3: Improved human resources management; Outcome 4: Improved governance and accountability; and Outcome 5: Improved regulation and quality assurance.

Institutions Reforms Act, 2015, which seeks to provide autonomy to the government-owned medical teaching institutions and their affiliated teaching hospitals to improve their performance in and responsiveness to the provision of quality health care services (see Chapter 2 for a detailed description of these key health sector policies and reforms).

In addition, the Government of Khyber Pakhtunkhwa launched a provincial social health protection initiative (SHPI) called the **Sehat Sahulat Program** in December 2015. The current reach of the program stands at 51% of the Khyber Pakhtunkhwa population and is being scaled up to 69%. The present benefit package provides 100% coverage for maternity care and cancer in the outpatient department (OPD), as well as all illnesses requiring hospitalization in secondary care hospitals and limited tertiary cover.[15] The **Khyber Pakhtunkhwa Health Roadmap**, which was launched in 2016, is an initiative that seeks to carry out targeted interventions in critical domains within the health sector. As new initiatives are being launched, such as management and operation of health facilities through public–private partnerships (PPPs), a contract management unit has been established to ensure efficient allocation of resources and effective collaboration between public and private entities. A health sector reforms unit was founded in 2014 to ensure that planned reforms are based on sound technical knowledge and to coordinate those reforms that have been undertaken. The health sector reforms unit is responsible for coming up with locally relevant solutions to the challenges faced by the province.

Furthermore, human resources for health (HRH) have been expanded through better incentives for medical staff. Overall, 3,000 new medical officers and other staff have been hired. Multiple health facilities at all levels are being renovated. The district health information system (DHIS) has been strengthened, and its quarterly reports are more regularly utilized to inform evidence-based decision-making as the reports provide disease patterns at health facilities and service utilization trends, among other information.

III.   Purpose and Scope

ADB has been providing technical and financial support to the health sector in Pakistan for the last 20 years. ADB's Operational Plan for Health, 2015–2020 identifies three key areas of investment for supporting the developing member countries to achieve universal health coverage (UHC). Upon the request of the Department of Health of Khyber Pakhtunkhwa, ADB commissioned this health sector review with a focus on (i) health governance, (ii) health infrastructure, and (iii) health financing.

The key objectives of the review were to identify bottlenecks and opportunities within the focus areas and to lay a foundation for the development of a sector-wide health plan. Although the review takes a broader view of the health sector, the key focus remains hospital care. For health governance, there is an emphasis on hospital autonomy and contracting. Within health infrastructure, the review looks at the status of physical and human resources, projections on demand for inpatient services, and quality of hospital care. Finally, the health financing section presents the current state and challenges according to specific health financing functions, including revenue collection, pooling, and purchasing, focusing on three critical elements of universal coverage, such as breadth, scope, and depth. Closely intertwined with health financing is public financial management (PFM), which plays a crucial role in ensuring that public funds

---

[15]   Sehat Sahulat Program. http://sehatsahulat.com.pk/.

provide sustainable financing. The PFM challenges are also presented for each of the health financing functions using the framework of the World Health Organization (WHO) in aligning PFM and health financing.[16] Each section ends with some recommendations moving forward.

IV. Methodology

The review began with a comprehensive desk review of current documents and data available from the DOH and allied offices. The review team, comprising ADB staff and international and national experts in governance, health facility planning, health financing, quality improvement, and behavior change communication, conducted a quantitative survey in secondary care hospitals with the support of Khyber Medical University. The facility survey covered 37 facilities including 6 teaching and specialized hospitals (1 private), 8 district headquarters (DHQ) hospitals (1 private) and 12 *tehsil* headquarters (THQ) hospitals, 3 other hospitals, 4 RHCs, and 4 other outpatient facilities. The survey aimed to shed additional light on the key governance and accountability issues identified in the HSS 2010–2017. During November 2017–February 2018, the ADB review team conducted two missions that involved detailed discussions with stakeholders—including more than 100 individuals from the DOH, allied offices, and government hospitals—and six on-site visits to secondary care hospitals.

After review and analysis of reports, statistics, and other documents, a questionnaire and a checklist were developed to guide the review visits at six selected secondary level hospitals.[17] The DOH purposively selected these 6 out of 97 secondary level hospitals in Khyber Pakhtunkhwa to represent a range of contexts in the province. Further, a team from the Khyber Medical University's faculty conducted a survey on both service performance in 7 out of 19 DHQ hospitals and the key referral structures at the district (secondary care) level.

---

[16] C. Cashin et al. 2017. Aligning Public Financial Management and Health Financing: Sustaining Progress Toward Universal Health Coverage. *Health Financing Working Paper*. No. 4. Geneva: WHO.

[17] Details on questionnaire developed and documents reviewed refer to M. Niechzial. 2018. *Challenges and Solutions for Better Quality*. Background paper for the Assessment of the Khyber Pakhtunkhwa Health Sector. Peshawar. 13–15 February.

CHAPTER 2
Health Governance

I. Overview

In sector and facility governance, reforms within Khyber Pakhtunkhwa have focused mostly on (i) providing managerial autonomy to tertiary hospitals or medical teaching institutions (MTIs) and, to a lesser extent, to other public health facilities; (ii) contracting out the provision of certain primary and secondary health services to private providers; and (iii) strengthening the health information systems such as the DHIS and health management information system (HMIS) for monitoring and evaluation (M&E) of health facilities.

While these reforms represent substantial advances toward strengthening the health system and improving its performance, fundamental weaknesses remain that can prevent or derail the implementation of these reforms or dilute their impact. This section looks at the health sector and health facilities governance and facility-level autonomy in Khyber Pakhtunkhwa as critical building blocks of the provincial health system.

II. Achievements

Health sector regulations in Khyber Pakhtunkhwa are quite comprehensive. Since 2011, more than 23 ordinances/acts and amendments about health care have been passed in Khyber Pakhtunkhwa. Some of these are novel and introduce new dimensions in terms of quality, access, and service delivery, while others, mostly amendments, seek to update the existing laws that are not in line with modern medical, scientific, or social standards. The most critical of these laws include the following:

- **Khyber Pakhtunkhwa Health Care Commission Act, 2015.** It aims to regulate the health care in the province through sound technical knowledge, resulting in the establishment of the HCC—a statutory body constituted in 2015 as a transformation from the previous Health Regulatory Authority to supervise both public and private health care providers— with multiple roles including (i) developing registration and licensing standards, (ii) establishing and enforcing minimum quality and safety standards, (iii) enhancing capacity of registered and licensed individuals, and (iv) imposing fees and fines. The HCC carries out these functions through multiple committees.
- **Khyber Pakhtunkhwa Public Health (Surveillance and Response) Ordinance, 2017.** Its goal is to implement measures that help prevent and control diseases. It creates a

public health committee whose key mandate is to comply with WHO's International Health Regulations (2005) and to ensure that adequate equipment for the requisite surveillance and monitoring is available.

- **Khyber Pakhtunkhwa Medical Teaching Institutions Reforms Act, 2015.** It seeks to provide autonomy to the government-owned MTIs and their affiliated teaching hospitals to improve their performance and responsiveness. This rather broad mandate is to be achieved through the formation of a board of governors for each medical institution. The roles and responsibilities of the board span over technical, financial, and policy domains. Furthermore, all medical colleges are to affiliate with Khyber Medical University (KMU). The act also elucidates the rules about the private practice of doctors within and outside the medical institutes.

Khyber Pakhtunkhwa undertook various initiatives toward universal health coverage. The following are just some of these initiatives:

- **Sehat Sahulat Program.** The Government of Khyber Pakhtunkhwa launched a social health protection initiative called the Sehat Sahulat Program in December 2015. The current reach of the program stands at 51% of the population of the province and is currently being scaled up to 69%. The three-phased program is enrolling households based on proxy means testing (PMT) at a PMT score of 16.7 in the first phase, 24.5 in the second, and 32.5 in the third.[18] The current benefit package provides limited tertiary cover and 100% coverage for maternity care, cancer in the OPD, and all illnesses requiring hospitalization in secondary care hospitals. However, with competing programs in place—especially vertical programs on diabetes, hepatitis, cancer, and HIV/AIDS—there is a confusion in the scope of programs, which will likely result in inefficient utilization of resources.
- **Independent monitoring unit.** An independent monitoring unit (IMU) has been established to monitor and evaluate all public sector health care facilities. The IMU is expected to help facilitate optimal utilization of public health facilities and in making evidence-informed decisions.
- **Khyber Pakhtunkhwa Health Roadmap.** It was launched in 2016 as an initiative to carry out targeted interventions in critical domains within health. These interventions include ensuring that adequate frontline staff and medicines are available, routine immunization of children is conducted, and regular data are generated with an emphasis on reliability. The Minister of Health reviews progress every 2 months in stocktake meetings with support from the IMU and road map team.
- **Public–private partnerships.** The previous PPP initiatives were criticized for poor management of contracts. As new initiatives are being launched—such as management and operation of health facilities through PPPs—a contract management unit has been created to guarantee efficient allocation of resources and effective collaboration between public and private entities.

---

[18] Indicators used for PMT scoring: (i) number of people in the household under the age of 18 or over the age of 65; (ii) highest education level of the household head; (iii) number of children in the household between 5 and 16 years old currently attending school; (iv) number of rooms per person; (v) type of toilet used by the household; (vi) at least one refrigerator, freezer, or washing machine; (vii) at least one air conditioner, air cooler, geyser, or heater; (viii) at least one cookstove, cooking range, or microwave oven; (ix) ownership of engine drive vehicles; (x) at least one TV; (xi) ownership of livestock; and (xii) ownership of agricultural land. The aforementioned indicators were developed using Pakistan Social and Living Standards Measurement data from 2005 to 2006.

- **Health sector reforms unit.** It was established in 2004 to ensure that planned reforms are based on sound technical knowledge and to coordinate the ones that have been undertaken. It is responsible for developing locally relevant solutions to the challenges faced by the province.
- **Human resources for health.** It has been expanded through better incentives for medical staff. Overall, 3,000 new medical officers and other staff have been hired, multiple health facilities at all levels are being renovated, and the DHIS has been strengthened and is now being more regularly utilized with quarterly reports from the department. These reports form the basis of decision-making as they provide, among other things, disease patterns at health facilities and service utilization trends.

III. Challenges

Documents and reports revealed several governance-related challenges in the Khyber Pakhtunkhwa health sector. Key governance and accountability issues identified in the HSS 2010–2017 include (i) inadequate emphasis on stewardship functions, (ii) lack of results-based decision-making, (iii) lack of clear financing and delivery strategies, (iv) poor health facility management, (v) weak capacity to deliver on new roles or functions, and (vi) inadequate financial accountability and internal controls. ADB surveyed health facilities to shed additional light on these issues. This section summarizes the findings from the survey and the documents and literature.

In analyzing governance challenges, this section used WHO's recommendation to focus on four areas within governance: (i) institutional design of the health sector, (ii) health policies, (iii) health regulations, and (iv) oversight and accountability (Figure 1). We then analyzed governance at the level of health facilities, with a special focus on hospital autonomy.

Figure 1: World Health Organization´s Dimensions of Health Sector Governance

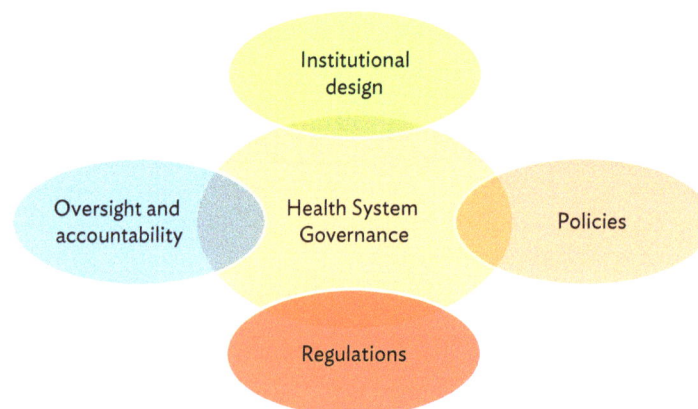

Source: Author's elaboration based on World Health Organization. 2010. *Health Systems Governance.* Geneva.

Regulations lacking consistency over time and clear linkages to health policies. Some legislative pieces have been issued in a clear effort to better define the regulatory framework for health in Khyber Pakhtunkhwa. Although comprehensive, the regulatory framework is yet to be implemented in most cases. Furthermore, important gaps remain, especially regarding service contracting and health PPPs (there is one general act on PPPs in Khyber Pakhtunkhwa but none focusing on health). In many cases, these regulations are not followed or supported by operational rules or an action plan. As a result, units and staff responsible for the application of these regulations have enormous difficulties in moving ahead and operationalizing them. The following are crucial issues that reduce the effectiveness of health regulations in Khyber Pakhtunkhwa and contribute to health system weaknesses.

System Fragmentation

First, legislation has promoted different waves and designs for decentralization over time (2001, 2012–2013), which in turn have contributed to system fragmentation and overlapping of responsibilities. Under the Khyber Pakhtunkhwa Local Government Act, 2013, the management and operation of basic health units (BHUs), RHCs, hospitals other than DHQs, and public health activities is devolved to local governments, while DHQs and teaching and tertiary facilities remain under the DOH. However, it is not clear which local government level (districts, *tehsils*, villages) will be responsible for which level of facilities, or more generally which health-related responsibilities are devolved to which local government level (this may contribute to the diversity of situations observed in the facility report on authority lines as shown in Table 1). On the other hand, a decentralized design has not taken due consideration of the managerial and technical capacity at the different levels of government: while district authorities struggle to meet their responsibilities, it is unclear what *tehsils*, village councils, and neighboring councils can effectively do in the health system except perhaps execute community-based services.

Second, existing regulations are often fragmented among various stakeholders and not fully consistent. They often focus on specific areas or challenges and lack a comprehensive framework that would align them to greater strategic goals. For example, regarding drug regulation, following an ineffective decentralization to provincial governments, the Ministry of National Health Services, Regulations and Coordination (NHSRC) is responsible for producer licensing, drug testing, drug registration, pricing, and trade through the Drug Regulatory Authority of Pakistan. The DOH, through its drug quality control boards, remains responsible for market surveillance, and the interim Pakistan Medical and Dental Council and the Pharmacy Council of Pakistan are responsible for licensing medical and pharmacy schools and practitioners.[19] Overall, 12 different regulations govern drug production, distribution, and use.

Inconsistent Enforcement

Third, regulations are not systematically enforced due to the insufficiency of qualified staff or the absence of mechanisms for doing so. For example, there is evidence that contracts are difficult to implement, as legislations do not provide a clear framework for it. Enforcement of drug regulation is hampered by insufficient staff (less than 50% of sanctioned posts are filled) (footnote 19).

Regulatory Voids

Fourth, some regulatory voids remain. The private health sector is mostly unregulated, although the HCC is initiating a process of mapping and monitoring the quality of service and accreditation of the private sector providers. However, the HCC lacks clarity on how to proceed and the necessary

---

[19] I. Nasir. 2018. *Drug Regulation*. Background paper for the Assessment of the Khyber Pakhtunkhwa Health Sector. Peshawar. 13–15 February.

staff and tools to do so. Health care quality is also marginally regulated. No comprehensive accreditation or quality assurance system is in place, and initiatives in the area tend to be isolated and focused. No standard operating procedures (SOPs) or clinical guidelines are available or used (footnote 17). The HCC has a critical role but has yet to develop an operational plan and lacks the necessary staff. Finally, the role of politically sensitive reforms such as PPPs and contracting out is unclear and requires a comprehensive health-specific regulatory framework. On the other hand, most of the new regulatory bodies lack sufficient qualified staff, which prevents them from effectively developing or enforcing appropriate health regulations. Some of the offices—including the Health Foundation, the HCC, and health reform unit—have few technical staff.

Structured but fragmented institutional design. The health sector in Khyber Pakhtunkhwa is composed of two broad subsectors: (i) the public sector, made of facilities operated by the provincial and local governments and structured by the level of care; and (ii) the private sector. OPD preventive services and a limited number of curative services are offered by all of these facilities, in contrast RHCs provide a wider range of curative services. In addition, outreach preventive services are offered by primary health care (PHC) facilities through vaccinators, sanitary patrol, and sanitary inspectors. DHQ, THQ, and civil hospitals provide highly specialized secondary health care, while teaching hospitals form the tertiary level. The institutional design of the health sector is greatly affected by the level and form of decentralization. Since the 18th Constitutional Amendment of 2010, responsibilities for health service delivery, among other functions, have been devolved to the provinces; devolution was further taken to the local governments by the Local Government Act, 2013. Altogether, there are 14 tertiary hospitals and 24 specialized hospitals, 199 secondary hospitals, and 1,471 PHC facilities (Table 1).

Complex Institutional Design
The provincial DOH, headed by the secretary health, is responsible for the design of health policies and strategies as well as M&E. It oversees three main units: (i) the health secretariat under the DOH, headed by the secretary health, supervises the sector coordination and delivery of tertiary and some secondary (DHQs) health care services including teaching medical institutions; (ii) the director general of health services coordinates various programs and district health service delivery and directs their implementation; and (iii) the health services academy manages in-service and pre-service training. The district health officers (DHOs) organize and deliver primary and secondary health services, except for the DHQ hospitals. The DHQs are monitored by the medical superintendents, reporting directly to the director general of health services.

Newly established units or bodies are in charge of policy and oversight functions: health sector reforms unit (reform strategies and initiatives), health financing (health insurance scheme), HCC (regulation and quality assurance), and IMU (M&E).

This decentralized system is further fragmented along subsectors (public, private, and donor-funded nongovernment organizations [NGOs]), and institutions (several departments involved in decision-making and resource allocation in health). DHOs provide primary health services and some hospital care (they operate THQ hospitals), while the DOH is formally responsible for secondary care but has little authority over the autonomous MTIs and a significant part of secondary care (it operates the DHQ hospitals). The DOH still focuses on direct service provision and is in the process of strengthening its coordination and stewardship role.

Table 1: Health Facility Network

Type of Facility	No. of Facilities	No. of Beds	Avg size
Tertiary and secondary care			
Category A hospitals, MTIs and non-MTIs	14	9,200	657
Specialized hospitals	24	1,604	67
District headquarter (DHQ) hospitals	19		
Tehsil headquarter (THQ) hospitals	78		
Category B	13	3,104	239
Category C	26	3,061	117
Category D	63		
Other (police)		150	
Primary care			
Rural health centers (RHCs)	111	1,324	12
Basic health units (BHUs)	776		
Civil dispensaries	446		
Mother and child health centers	49		
Sub-health centers, TB and leprosy clinics	89		
All facilities	1,708	18,433	

TB= tuberculosis, MTI= medical teaching institution.

Source: Government of Khyber Pakhtunkhwa, Department of Health. 2017.

Various health subsystems coexist that are managed by separate organizations: (i) DOH (for tertiary and some secondary care); (ii) local governments (for primary care and most secondary care); (iii) armed forces; and (iv) various independent health insurance schemes including (i) SHPI[20] (operated by State Life Insurance Corporation of Pakistan [SLIC]), (ii) Employees Social Security Institution for public servants, (iii) Zakat and Bait-ul-Mal funds (funded by household contributions), and (iv) several private insurance organizations. Little coordination takes place between these different subsystems. Although the DOH and DHOs operate health facilities in the same district (e.g., DHQ hospitals), catering to the same population, there is no system for joint health planning and budgeting or coordinated supervision at the district level.

This fragmentation tends to prevent the integration and coordination among the various subsectors and also blurs authority and accountability lines. The facility survey undertaken for this review illustrates this lack of clarity in authority lines and responsibilities; most facilities (70%)

---

[20] H. Huitzing. 2018. *Actuarial Model for the Supply and Demand Side Interventions in the Khyber Pakhtunkhwa Health Sector.* Background paper for the Assessment of the Khyber Pakhtunkhwa Health Sector. Peshawar. 13–15 February.

report being under the management of the provincial government (DOH), irrespective of the level and type of facility (Table 2), including 83% of THQs and 50% of PHC facilities (which are formally under the management of the DHOs). On the other hand, two tertiary-level hospitals, which are under the provincial management, report to the DHOs.

The distribution of general managerial authority does not necessarily match the responsibilities for specific functions: 22% of facilities report having staff salaries paid by the Department of Finance, while the rest are paid by either the DOH or through donor assistance (for one facility only). Similar variations are found for payments made for medical supplies and drugs and other operational expenses (Table 3). It is unclear whether these conflicting views are due to actual variation in allocation of responsibilities, the lack of clarity in authority lines, or poor information at the facility level. Coordination between the DOH and DHOs is inadequate, as no consolidated district-level planning or budgeting mechanism is in place. The roles of the facility and district levels appear to be more overlapping than complementary. In any case, these perceptions reflect the blurred distribution of authority and responsibilities. The responsibility of paying for inputs in private facilities is clearer and relies on the private owner of the facility.

Table 2: Authority Lines and Responsibilities for Health Facilities

Facility Type	Provincial DOH	District Health	Private	Total
Teaching hospitals	1	1		2
Specialized hospitals	2	1	1	4
DHQ hospitals	7		1	8
THQ hospitals	10	2		12
Other hospitals	2	1		3
RHCs	1	3		4
Dispensaries		1		1
Mother and child health centers	1			1
Other outpatient facilities	2			2
Total	**26**	**9**	**2**	**37**

DHQ = district headquarters, DOH = Department of Health, RHC = rural health center, THQ = *tehsil* headquarters.

Source: Khyber Medical University, Health Facility Survey, 2017.

Table 3: Distribution of Selected Payment Responsibilities across Public Facilities

Facility Type	Staff Salaries			Medical Supplies			Other Operations		
Responsibility	DOH	DOF	DA	DOH	DOF	DA	DOH	DOF	DA
Teaching hospitals		2			1	1		1	1
Specialized hospitals	1	1	1	2	1		2	1	1
DHQ hospitals	6	1		6	1		6	1	
THQ hospitals	9	3		10	1	1	9	1	2
Other hospitals	2	1		2		1	2		1
RHC	4			3		1	3		1
Civil dispensary	1			1			1		
Mother and child health centers	1			1			1		
Other outpatient facilities	2			2			2		
Total	26	8	1	27	4	4	26	4	6

DA = donor assistance, DHQ = district headquarters, DOF = Department of Finance, DOH = Department of Health, RHC = rural health center, THQ = *tehsil* headquarters.

Source: Khyber Medical University, Health Facility Survey, 2017.

A robust but incomplete policy framework. Many health sector policies have been developed, but important challenges remain. First, no comprehensive and clear reform agenda is in place. The HSS 2010–2017 has yet to be updated to specifically include several reform efforts of recent years, although more recently the DOH has already initiated the update process. The reform initiatives need to be aligned under this updated HSS as a comprehensive reform agenda that sets long-term objectives and coordinates them effectively. Second, reform initiatives are sparsely documented. Limited evidence is available on the impact of these innovative models. Few rigorous evaluations of these experiences have been conducted. These evaluations have been challenged on various grounds, and some of them have been discontinued without a clear technical rationale. No M&E system allows for a rigorous review of past and current reform experiences, which prevents learning.

A preliminary assessment—to be confirmed by meticulous documentation—of these experiences suggests that at least some of these reform initiatives have been successful at improving management processes, quality, and efficiency, and have been discontinued for reasons unrelated to their actual performance. Reasons for success include management stability, managerial autonomy, and technical capacity of new managers. Some of the reasons for the lack of continuity in these innovative efforts relate to unsustained political support and interest, lack of capacity for contract management and M&E on the contracting side (usually the DOH), and end-of-the-project funding by the donors involved.

Poor accountability mechanisms. At the sector level, coordination with international donors is done through the Sectoral Coordination Committee, which is chaired by the secretary health and the representative of the Department for International Development of the United Kingdom and includes five DOH staff and representatives of key donors as members. The committee has been instrumental in mapping donors´ support and the remaining gaps. However, the committee has met irregularly and is not fully effective in ensuring complementarity and avoiding duplications in donor assistance.

Accountability mechanisms have been strengthened since 2014 with the establishment of the IMU (which monitors a series of key performance indicators), financial management cell, procurement cell, internal audit, and district-level health management committees. Again, these initiatives are too recent to have a clear impact. Many of these new units struggle to move forward with their responsibilities due to limited numbers of qualified staff and the lack of clear guidance on how to operationalize these new functions. The introduction of output-based budgeting in 2010 aims at linking budget allocation with clear program goals and targets. However, given the challenges facing planning and budget preparation, the effectiveness of this innovation to promote efficiency and accountability is still unclear.[21]

Unclear roles and responsibilities and weak and unsystematic guidance and support from the Department of Health and the Donor Assistance. Facility managers are mostly physicians who spend some of their time, or take a leave from their physician duties, to supervise the facility. They are not trained in or familiarized with management objectives, principles, or tools. Furthermore, given the systematic underfunding and lack of agreed process or management guidelines, they spend most of their time attending to "issues" requiring their immediate attention rather than planning and managing organized processes. There are no monitoring, feedback, or review mechanisms for key performance and quality indicators that can aid in better management of the facilities.

Aside from the small number of qualified managerial staff, a big challenge lies in the absence of clear guidance and rules about the work process in the facilities. Processes for clinical and managerial activities are not standardized, and facility staff are by and large not bounded by any protocols in decision-making. Although an increasing number of standards and rules are being developed by the DOH, they have yet to find their way to the facility level. For example, hospital managers are often unaware of secondary health care standards, even though they are available. Quality assurance measures and patient flow guidelines are unavailable,[22] and field visits evidence a lot of improvisation in both clinical and managerial work processes.

While facility managers are supposed to prepare and submit their budget in a formally decentralized budgeting system, they are not trained on how to do so and have little knowledge of budget procedures or budget preparation. As a result, budget estimates prepared by facility managers are inconsistent and mostly incremental; the final approved budget, decided centrally, has little link to the sector or facility plans. There is widespread evidence of "non-compliance of delegation between authorities and requirements for proper documentation of expenditures, misclassification of expenditures and misuse of public funds and assets" (footnote 21).

---

[21] A. Mahmood. 2018. *Public Financial Management Assessment: Health Sector.* Background paper for the Assessment of the Khyber Pakhtunkhwa Health Sector. Peshawar. 13–15 February.

[22] This varies substantially across facility levels and management or ownership, as discussed above.

Coupled with weak and unsystematic guidance and support from the DOH and the donor assistance, many facilities, especially at the local level, appear to be left to themselves and to address only the most urgent needs of patients with little process standardization or supervision. However, it is worth noting that this picture varies greatly across facilities, with some succeeded in effecting some change and being managed in a much better fashion than the average. These situations appear to be linked to the stability of management and strong individual leadership.

Poor information systems. Existing information systems focus on reporting and monitoring the use of inputs and the production of specific services and do not emphasize efficiency, quality, and overall performance. The DOH has in recent years established an IMU to strengthen information systems, and this unit has been improving data collection and analysis on health service delivery. But performance and outcome indicators are still little used or collected, and capacity for interpreting these data is inadequate. The Government of Khyber Pakhtunkhwa has recently launched the e-Governance initiative that aims at making public service providers more accountable, but this is still in process and has yet to affect the health sector.

Political interference, weak oversight, and corrupt practices. Interference from local politicians or interest groups (such as political parties) on staff appointment and day-to-day operations is a constant practice especially at local health facilities and prevents effective management. On average, managers spend around 7 months in their position before being replaced, which is not enough for them to get familiar with the facility operation and challenges. Given the time constraints, it is quite difficult, if not impossible, for a facility manager to plan and implement effective managerial practices or interventions for strengthening facility operations, or even to implement national or provincial health policies. Furthermore, there is no incentive whatsoever for managers to pursue efficiency or quality goals, as managerial decisions tend to follow objectives unrelated to the good operation of the facilities themselves.

Political interference, weak oversight, poor information systems, and low managerial capacity at the local level contribute to the extension of unethical practices under different forms: informal payments to health professionals, high staff absenteeism, dual practice (public and private) from health professionals, nonqualified providers in the private sector, waste and loss of medical and other supplies, etc. Such practices tend to divert or waste essential and scarce resources from service provision, which is hard to measure; however, estimates range from at least 20% of world GDP (Organisation for Economic Co-operation and Development) to 25% (African Union). WHO estimates that 10%–25% of procurement expenses in health are lost to corruption, and an additional 10%–25% are wasted due to inefficiencies in resource allocation and use.[23]

Inconsistent political support for innovative models. Over the years, the Government of Khyber Pakhtunkhwa has contracted out the management and/or the provision of primary hospital services to various private organizations (usually NGOs or charity organizations). These contracts include the PPP arrangements with Aga Khan Foundation (and its Aga Khan Health Services)—the largest nonprofit organization in Pakistan—for the management of hospitals and PHC in the remote Chitral District. Aga Khan has similar arrangements in other provinces including Sindh, Baltistan, and Punjab. The contracts also include the People's Primary Healthcare Initiative (PPHI) experience. While systematic evaluations of these experiences have not been done, a few focused audit and assessment reports are available, and field visits can provide some insights. In spite of some limitations in the number, scope, and methodological design of some

---

[23] WHO. 2010. Chapter 4: More Health for the Money. In *The World Health Report: Health Systems Financing: The Path to Universal Coverage*. Geneva.

evaluations, available evidence suggests that these experiences of health PPPs or contracting out health service provision have been mostly successful. However, contracts are suspended for political reasons and due to the weaknesses in the contracting instrument. The prospects for further contracting out or increasing the autonomy of secondary hospitals are thus unclear, irrespective of technical arguments (see Appendix 1 for a case study on the hospital contracting experience in Khyber Pakhtunkhwa).

IV.   Recommendations

Given the past and current experience of the health sector in Khyber Pakhtunkhwa, strengthening the health sector and facility-level governance is a critical element of reform efforts. It involves addressing directly the structural challenges and weaknesses that have prevented change to take root and successful experiences to be replicated or expanded. While the Government of Khyber Pakhtunkhwa is working on some needed initiatives that contribute to strengthening the health sector and facility-level governance, the recommendations below focus on key elements that are missing and can bring together and align all these reform efforts and make them sustainable.

1.   **Strengthen institutional design: a clear vision and road map for the future.** Health reforms have largely been undertaken piecemeal, without a comprehensive vision for the health sector. Such a vision is fundamental for guiding current reforms, establishing transparent long-term goals, and ensuring coherence of different reform initiatives. The DOH needs to develop such a vision and a clear road map to get there. The current HSS 2010–2017 provides several elements but fails to bring together coherently the various reform initiatives. The long-term objectives and roles of PPP and hospital autonomy initiatives, among others, need to be clearly defined and aligned to ensure the continuity of purpose and avoid the launching of stand-alone projects that too often end with the project funding. As part of this vision, the governance structure of the health sector should be clarified and streamlined, including the roles and responsibilities of the DOH, donor assistance, facility boards, and facility management. Specific mechanisms to strengthen district-level coordination between DOH, donor assistance, and health facilities should be devised, such as a system for joint planning and budgeting and supervision structures and processes.

2.   **Strengthen the policy framework: a new approach to health facilities autonomy.** The recent experience on facility autonomy has meant "letting facilities manage themselves," without establishing clear mechanisms for M&E and performance assessment and without clarifying the role and authority of the DOH (as the sector steward) with regard to autonomous institutions. Hospital autonomy and PPP reforms need three critical elements to achieve their expected outcomes: (i) strong capacity on the contracting side (usually the DOH), (ii) strong contract between the DOH and the provider organization to ensure that the autonomous organization will actively pursue objectives aligned with health policies and priorities, and (iii) strong capacity at the facility management for modernizing management practices and improving quality and efficiency. In this view, it is critical to strengthen the technical and managerial capacity of facility managers and board members through rigorous training and the adoption of standard management and information tools and processes.

3. **Strengthen accountability: a new contracting framework.** A strong contractual arrangement is a critical piece to ensure that autonomy and PPP reforms deliver according to expectations. Such a contracting arrangement is nearly absent in the case of MTIs and weak in the case of outsourced health facilities. A contracting framework involves three critical elements: (i) a contracting entity with capacity for contract management and M&E, (ii) an implementing organization (public or private) with technical and managerial capacity and qualifications, and (iii) a contracting instrument (the contract itself) with certain required elements and features. While existing agreements have these three elements, the requisites for successfully managing contracts and achieving the expected results are not truly present. First, the contracting organization, usually the DOH (but also insurers such as SLIC) do not have staff trained in contract management. M&E of contracts is also weak, and existing information systems are not appropriate for contract management. The DOH has only recently established a central monitoring unit (CMU)and an IMU, and building their technical and financial capacity will require systematic training. Second, information on the private sector and potential partners or contractors is minimal. There is limited objective evidence of technical and financial capacity of individual providers, except for a few larger organizations. The DOH needs to start to systematically map private providers and gather relevant information on their capacity and features. Finally, the contracting instrument is either missing (e.g., in the case of MTIs) or weak. Several suspensions of existing contracts can be traced to weaknesses in the contract itself, including unclear objectives and goals, or undefined criteria for measuring compliance and performance (see Appendix 2 for the key elements of a strong contract). The DOH will increasingly need to monitor and evaluate provider contracts and more specifically providers´ performance, both for public and private facilities. To properly measure facility performance—which in turn should be reflected in the amount of payment as mentioned above—existing information systems (HMIS, DHIS) need to be revised to move their main focus from measuring inputs (staff, equipment, beds, expenditure) to measuring outcomes and results (achievement of agreed goals and targets, improvements in quality and efficiency).

4. **Strengthen regulations: address political interference and enforce contracts.** Evidence suggests that widespread political interference is likely to be the greatest challenge to health system efficiency and quality. The DOH should consider and assess various options for addressing the issue, including revising and enforcing legislation to prevent it, and outsourcing facility management and PPPs. The vision document proposed in recommendation no. 1 should reflect the findings of this review and define the key strategy or strategies to address it. Based on the review of experiences in Khyber Pakhtunkhwa made in this report, providing real autonomy to health facilities and contracting out their management (especially through PPP arrangements) are the most effective approach, but a more in-depth analysis is required to inform this critical discussion better. In addition, regulations should be revised to allow and support the enforcement of contracts. If this is not done, current and future contracts, especially those relating to innovative reforms, will not be enforced and will thus lose their potential to shape the future design of the health sector.

CHAPTER 3

Health Infrastructure

I. Overview

As discussed in earlier chapters, the Government of Khyber Pakhtunkhwa revitalized its health sector reform efforts with the HSS 2010–2017, the development of the essential health service packages for primary and secondary health care, and the secondary level minimum health services delivery package (MHSDP) for secondary care hospitals. In addition, the establishment of the HCC was another key step undertaken by the DOH to improve quality, safety, and efficiency of health care in the province.

Resource allocation is a fundamental component for effective service delivery, both in infrastructure and in trained health care professionals. This section reviews the current state of health service provision and human resources for health (HRH) in Khyber Pakhtunkhwa. Using a population growth-based adjusted model to predict the health service and HRH needs, the potential and relative gaps in resources to deliver health services through 2035 are enumerated across the districts. The section primarily focuses on hospital care, as this component of the health system constitutes a significant proportion (about 75%) of public resource allocations. Interspersed within the chapter is a discussion on the quality of care, which is at the core of health service delivery. The review pays special attention to the following factors (determinants) of quality: (i) infrastructure and equipment, (ii) utilization of inpatient and outpatient services, (iii) availability and functioning of key referral services, (iv) availability and functioning of crucial support services, and (v) quality of clinical care (analysis of patient records and interviews of clinical staff).

II. Achievements

To ensure equitable provision of quality health care services to all Khyber Pakhtunkhwa residents, the province has taken on developing minimum service delivery standards through MHSDP for primary health care facilities reports and secondary level MHSDP for secondary care hospitals.[24]

---

[24] A. Faisel. 2012. *Minimum Health Services Delivery Package for Primary Health Care Facilities in Khyber Pakhtunkhwa;* I. Thaver and M. Khalid. 2016. *Final Report: Secondary Level Minimum Health Services Delivery Package for Secondary Care Hospitals (MHSDP).*

The MHSDP reports provide a framework for primary and secondary health services from the perspective of service provision, infrastructure, human resources, equipment and supplies, and other system service considerations. Broadly, it defines the following:

- Dispensaries: provide 6-hour general treatment services, antenatal and postnatal services, immunization services, and limited health education services.
- Basic health units (BHUs): provide 6-hour planned health education services at the center and schools; general treatment services; antenatal, delivery, and postnatal services; limited laboratory services; and referral services.
- Rural health centers (RHCs): provide 6-hour planned health education services at the center and schools, general treatment services, selected surgical and minor procedural services, 24-hour delivery and newborn care, medicolegal services, inpatient services, emergency and urgent care services, and referral services.
- Category A, secondary hospitals: should have 350 inpatient beds, 6 dialysis units, 6 dentistry units, serving inpatient and outpatient services. Clinical specialties are surgery; medicine; gynecology/obstetrics; pediatrics; eye; ear, nose, throat (ENT); orthopedics; cardiology; psychiatry; chest/tuberculosis; dialysis unit, dentistry unit; pediatric surgery; neurosurgery; dermatology; accident and emergency (A&E); intensive care unit (ICU); and pediatric nursery/ICU. The target catchment area is around 1 million.
- Category B, secondary hospitals: should have 210 inpatient beds, 4 dialysis units, 4 dentistry units, serving inpatient and outpatient services. Clinical specialties are surgery, medicine, gynecology/obstetrics, pediatrics, eye, ENT, orthopedics, cardiology, psychiatry, chest/tuberculosis, dialysis unit, dentistry unit, A&E, ICU, and pediatric nursery/ICU. The target catchment area is around 500,000.
- Category C, secondary hospitals: should have 110 inpatient beds, 2 dentistry units, serving inpatient and outpatient services. Clinical specialties are surgery, medicine, gynecology/obstetrics, pediatric medicine, eye, ENT, orthopedics, A&E department (previously known as "casualty"), and ICU. The target catchment area is around 300,000.
- Category D, secondary hospitals: should have 40 inpatient beds, 1 dentistry unit, serving inpatient and outpatient services. Clinical specialties are surgery, medicine, gynecology/obstetrics, pediatric medicine, and A&E department. The target catchment area is around 100,000.

III.   Current Status

Public sector facilities are composed of hospitals ranging from MTIs to secondary and district-level hospitals (also known as district headquarters [DHQ] hospitals and public hospitals) and supported by RHCs.[25] These facility types have inpatient bed capacities and are further supported by a range of un-bedded facilities: BHUs, government rural dispensaries, mother and child health centers, and tuberculosis clinics (Figure 2). See Appendix 3 for a map of the distribution of public health facilities.

While the private sector exists in Khyber Pakhtunkhwa, the government is the main provider of preventive care throughout the province and the major provider of curative services in rural areas. The private sector is made up of a range of providers from reputable hospitals to unregistered single-operator quacks. Accurate numbers of facilities, bed numbers, and volume of services

---

[25] Government of Khyber Pakhtunkhwa, DOH, Notification no. 6-39/Notification/SPO/PC/H/VOL.

Figure 2: Public Health Facilities by Hierarchy of Service Provision

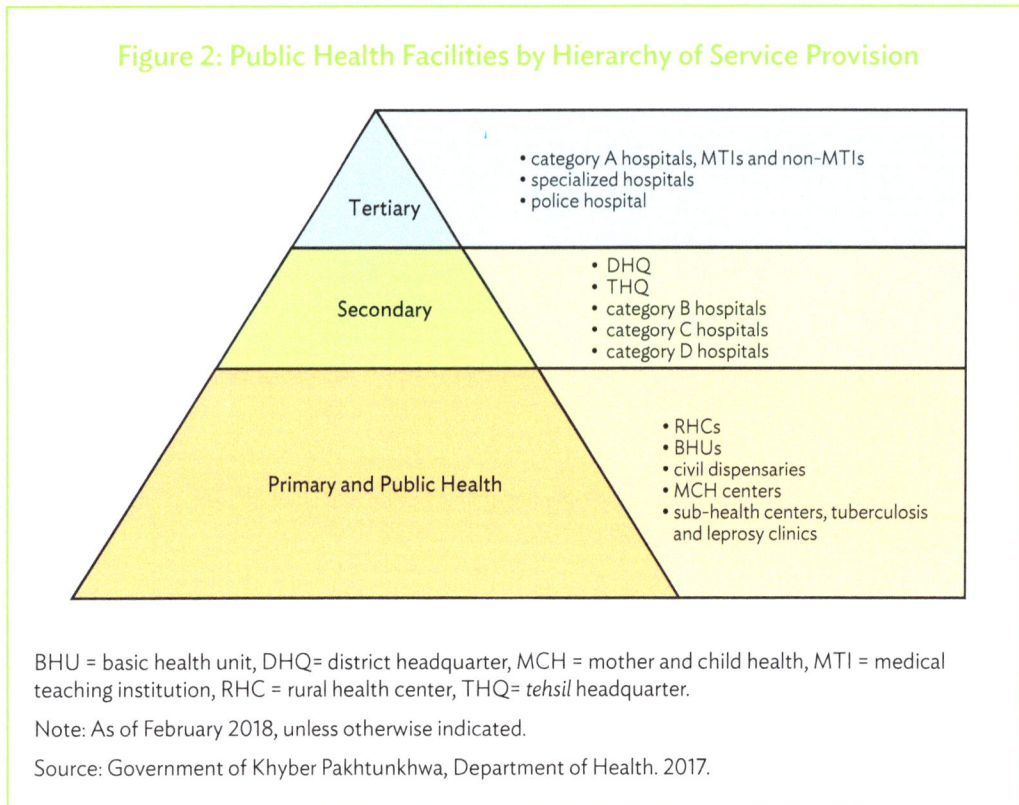

Tertiary
- category A hospitals, MTIs and non-MTIs
- specialized hospitals
- police hospital

Secondary
- DHQ
- THQ
- category B hospitals
- category C hospitals
- category D hospitals

Primary and Public Health
- RHCs
- BHUs
- civil dispensaries
- MCH centers
- sub-health centers, tuberculosis and leprosy clinics

BHU = basic health unit, DHQ= district headquarter, MCH = mother and child health, MTI = medical teaching institution, RHC = rural health center, THQ= *tehsil* headquarter.

Note: As of February 2018, unless otherwise indicated.

Source: Government of Khyber Pakhtunkhwa, Department of Health. 2017.

provided are unknown, although ministry officials estimate that the private sector delivers 40% of outpatient care and 10% of inpatient care from a range of facility types such as hospitals, clinics, centers, and dispensaries. Accurate capacity and infrastructure information on the private sector is not readily available due to the paucity of data reported and lack of information shared between public and private systems, although there are now attempts to begin registering private health care providers through the HCC.

Primary and community health services across Khyber Pakhtunkhwa are delivered from a combination of facilities consisting of smaller hospitals, dispensaries, RHCs, tuberculosis clinics, mother and child health centers, sub-health centers, BHUs, and leprosy clinics. Distribution of dispensaries and BHUs is based on population centers, and the provision of RHCs is dependent on the remoteness of the population and distance to reach secondary care hospitals. This issue is demonstrated by the relatively low provision of RHCs in more highly populated districts such as Abbottabad, Bannu, Charsadda, Dera Ismail Khan, Mardan, and Swat. There is no provision of RHCs in Peshawar District. An outlay of the providers in public and private health care systems is presented in Figure 3.

Hospital beds. By proportion of population served, bed numbers are relatively well distributed across the districts, except Peshawar and Abbottabad, which have markedly higher bed capacity than the proportion of population. The districts of Charsadda, Mansehra, Mardan, Swabi, and Swat have noticeably lower bed capacity than the proportion of population. The number of hospital beds per 10,000 population for Khyber Pakhtunkhwa demonstrates a relatively consistent trend for the province compared with overall Pakistan at 6 beds per 10,000 population in the most

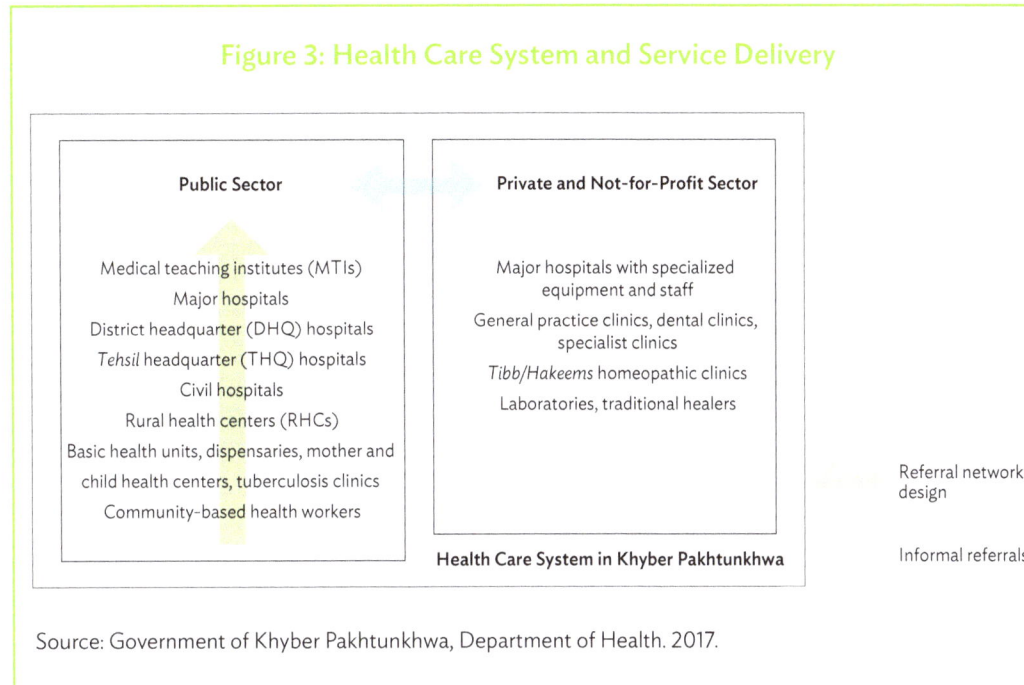

Figure 3: Health Care System and Service Delivery

Public Sector

Medical teaching institutes (MTIs)
Major hospitals
District headquarter (DHQ) hospitals
Tehsil headquarter (THQ) hospitals
Civil hospitals
Rural health centers (RHCs)
Basic health units, dispensaries, mother and child health centers, tuberculosis clinics
Community-based health workers

Private and Not-for-Profit Sector

Major hospitals with specialized equipment and staff
General practice clinics, dental clinics, specialist clinics
Tibb/Hakeems homeopathic clinics
Laboratories, traditional healers

Health Care System in Khyber Pakhtunkhwa

Referral network design

Informal referrals

Source: Government of Khyber Pakhtunkhwa, Department of Health. 2017.

recent indicators reported (five for Afghanistan and seven for India, its neighboring countries).[26] The number of beds per 10,000 population across Khyber Pakhtunkhwa has remained relatively consistent over the last 8 years, peaking in 2012 at 6.21 hospital beds (both public and private).

Renal dialysis. Renal dialysis services and capacity in Khyber Pakhtunkhwa are not well known. The Kidney Foundation of the National Institute of Kidney and Urological Diseases last reported a registry in 2014, listing three facilities in the province (one in Mardan and two in Peshawar) with 34 dialysis machines servicing 335 patients.[27] Based on the bed capacity descriptions of secondary care hospitals from the MHSDP and estimates of secondary care hospitals, there are up to 84 dialysis machines in category A hospitals across the province and 52 machines in category B hospitals (footnote 27).

Medical practitioners. The government employed 3,644 medical practitioners, 10 radiologists, and an additional 122 dental surgeons in 2016.[28] The private sector has 5,075 medical practitioners registered in 2016, 90.8% of whom are males with 466 (9.2%) females. The ratio of government-employed doctors to population shows that filled medical posts are relatively well distributed across all districts, except Dera Ismail Khan, Bannu, and Charsadda with a notably lower ratio, and Swat, Karak, and Haripur with a higher ratio (Figure 4). The rate of doctors per 1,000 population for Khyber Pakhtunkhwa is low at 0.3 doctors (in the public and private sector) compared with

---

[26] World Bank. Hospital beds (per 1,000 people). https://data.worldbank.org/indicator/SH.MED.BEDS.ZS (accessed 10 January 2018).

[27] The Kidney Foundation. 2014. *Dialysis Registry of Pakistan, 2014*. http://www.kidneyfoundation.net.pk/KF_Book.pdf.

[28] Government of Khyber Pakhtunkhwa, Planning and Development Department, Bureau of Statistics. 2017. *Development Statistics of Khyber Pakhtunkhwa, 2017*. Pakistan.

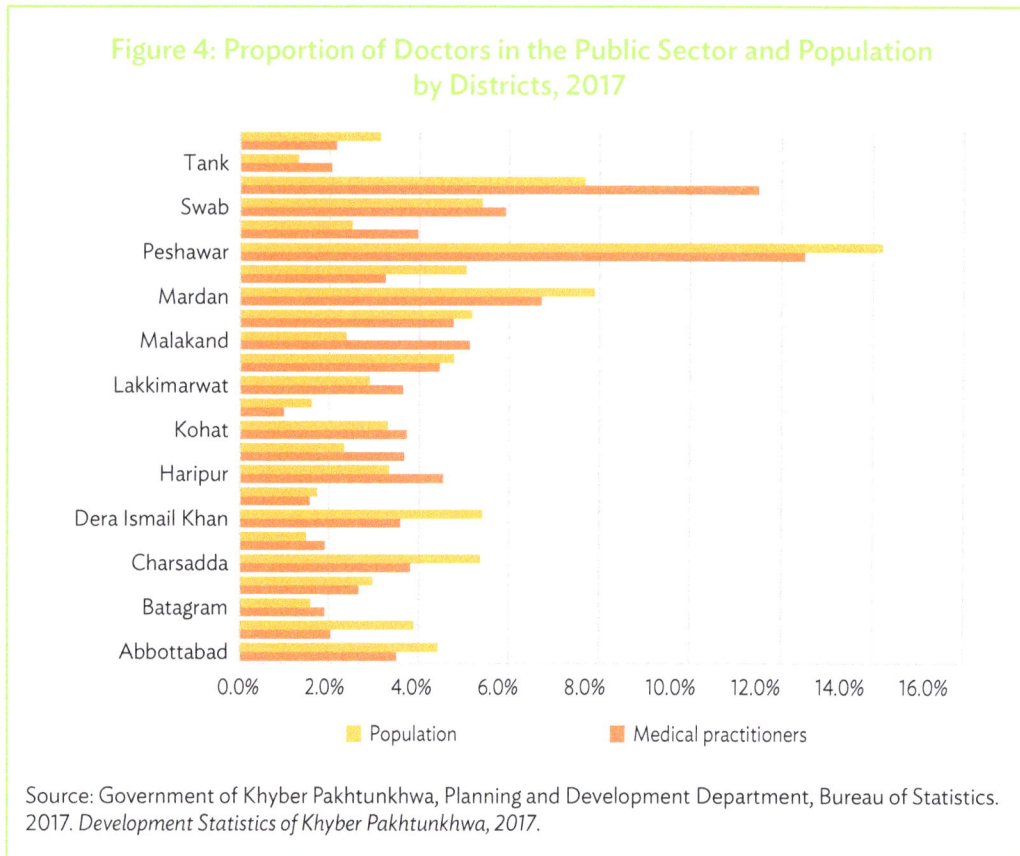

Figure 4: Proportion of Doctors in the Public Sector and Population by Districts, 2017

Source: Government of Khyber Pakhtunkhwa, Planning and Development Department, Bureau of Statistics. 2017. *Development Statistics of Khyber Pakhtunkhwa, 2017.*

overall Pakistan at 0.8 doctors in the most recent countrywide indicators; the rate is 0.3 doctors in Afghanistan and 0.7 doctors in India per 1,000 population.[29]

Nurses. The DOH has over 6,000 posts for nursing staff across Khyber Pakhtunkhwa, with a vacancy rate of 10% in November 2017, as reported by interviews with the DOH management personnel.[30] In terms of government hospital beds by districts, nursing posts are relatively well distributed across the province, except for Peshawar, which has a significantly greater nurse-to-population ratio than other districts, and Kohistan and Charsadda, which have noticeably lower nurse-to-population ratio (Figure 5). The number of nurses per 10,000 population for the province is low at 2.0 nurses compared with overall Pakistan at 6.0 nurses in the most recent indicators (3.6 nurses for Afghanistan and 20.5 nurses for India).[31] This difference between Khyber Pakhtunkhwa and Pakistan may be due to the unknown number of registered nurses practicing in the private sector, which is regulated by the Pakistan Nursing Council, a national licensing and registration authority.

---

[29] World Bank. Physicians (per 1,000 people). https://data.worldbank.org/indicator/SH.MED.PHYS.ZS (accessed 10 January 2018).

[30] Government of Khyber Pakhtunkhwa, DOH. Sanctioned Posts of Charge Nurses, Head Nurses, Nursing Instructor/ Nursing Superintendent, and Chief Nursing Superintendent/Vice Principal/Nursing Instructor Lists. Unpublished.

[31] World Bank. Nurses and Midwives (per 1,000 people). https://data.worldbank.org/indicator/SH.MED.NUMW.P3 (accessed 10 January 2018).

Figure 5: Proportion of Nurses in the Public Sector and Population by Districts, 2017

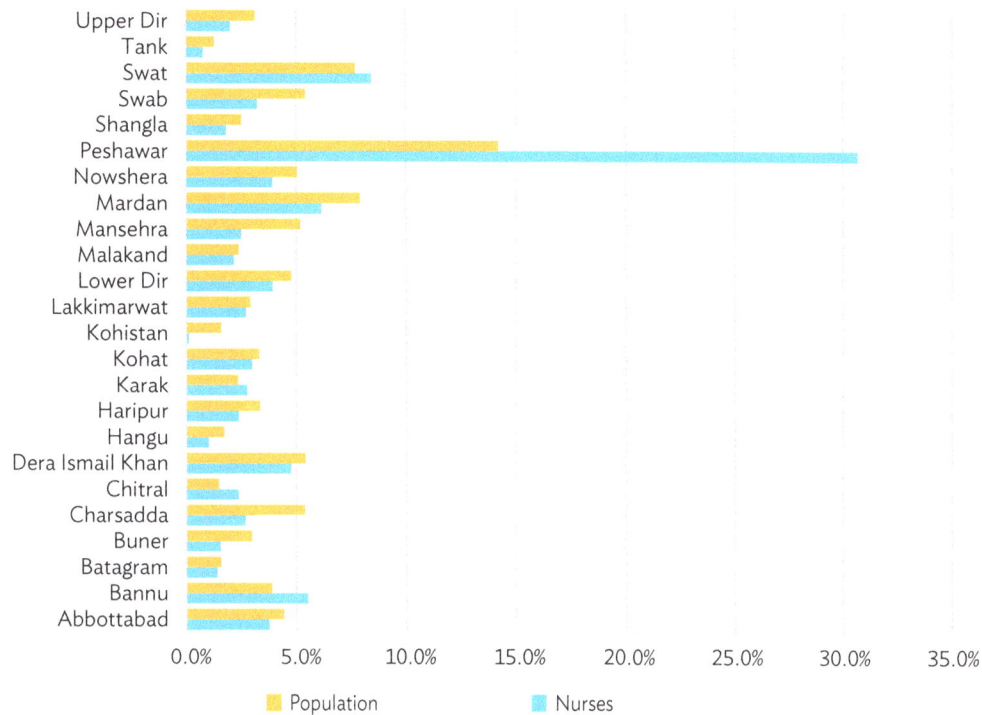

Source: Government of Khyber Pakhtunkhwa, Department of Health. 2017.

Inpatient care provision. According to the recent discussions with the DOH and executive managers of MTIs, approximately 350,000 admissions annually were made in MTIs in recent years, and the private sector has been providing 10% of all inpatient requirements.[32] The Lady Reading Hospital in Peshawar alone, the largest MTI in Khyber Pakhtunkhwa, contributes to approximately 150,000 admissions per year.[33] Based on these data, about 930,000 patients were admitted and treated within hospitals in 2015. The estimated rate of inpatient admissions for the Khyber Pakhtunkhwa population in 2015 is 32.5 admissions per 1,000 population (Table 4), which is significantly lower than other countries; for example the discharge rate is 133 per 1,000 population in Kyrgyzstan and 111 in Tajikistan.[34]

[32] S. G. Khan, chief planning officer, Department of Health, Khyber Pakhtunkhwa, personal communication, 14 February 2018.

[33] M. Zaman, medical director, Lady Reading Hospital Peshawar, personal communication, 14 February 2018.

[34] Organisation for Economic Co-operation and Development. Hospital discharge rates. https://data.oecd.org/healthcare/hospital-discharge-rates.htm (accessed on 11 January 2018).

Table 4: Inpatient Admission per 1,000 Population, 2009–2015

	2009	2010	2011	2012	2013	2014	2015
Estimated total inpatient admissions	391,278	553,111	886,971	835,848	573,403	823,191	932,029
Population (thousand)	24,307	24,993	25,697	26,421	27,166	27,932	28,721
Admission per 1,000 population	16.10	22.13	34.52	31.64	21.11	29.47	32.45

Source: Government of Khyber Pakhtunkhwa, Department of Health. 2017.

Outpatient and ambulatory care. The number of district-level patients treated in the outpatient setting as published in the Development Statistics indicates a rapidly growing trend of patients seeking outpatient services from government facilities, excluding the MTIs, with year-on-year growth reported between 2011 and 2015 and an average annual growth rate of 54% over the last 6 years. The estimated outpatient consultations for Khyber Pakhtunkhwa as a rate of the population demonstrates a growing trend of annual physician visits per capita from 0.72 consultations per person in 2009 to 2.5 by 2015, a rate still lower than comparable countries which is 3.5 for Kyrgyzstan and 4.5 in Tajikistan.

Table 5: Outpatient Visits per Capita, 2009–2015

	2009	2010	2011	2012	2013	2014	2015
Estimated total outpatient consultations	17,448,222	22,316,084	18,043,728	43,753,003	49,596,128	60,019,347	72,275,272
Population (thousand)	24,307	24,993	25,697	26,421	27,166	27,932	28,721
Outpatient visit per capita	0.72	0.89	0.70	1.66	1.83	2.15	2.52

Source: Government of Khyber Pakhtunkhwa, Department of Health. 2017.

IV.   Challenges

Unmet demand for inpatient and outpatient care. The modeled estimate indicates that 1.7 million inpatient admissions will be required across the province by 2020, growing to 3.1 million by 2035. The demand for acute services, converted to hospital beds, demonstrates an overall increasing trend from 22,100 beds in 2020 to 39,200 beds by 2035, equivalent to an average demand growth rate of approximately 5.1% per annum. Comparison of modeled requirements to current service provision shows a current and prevailing gap in acute hospital services province-wide. In 2015, this gap was calculated to be an undersupply of almost 460,000 inpatient admissions. By 2020, without further investment in service provision and infrastructure, the gap will grow to 752,000 patient admissions, increasing to a gap of almost 2.2 million patients by

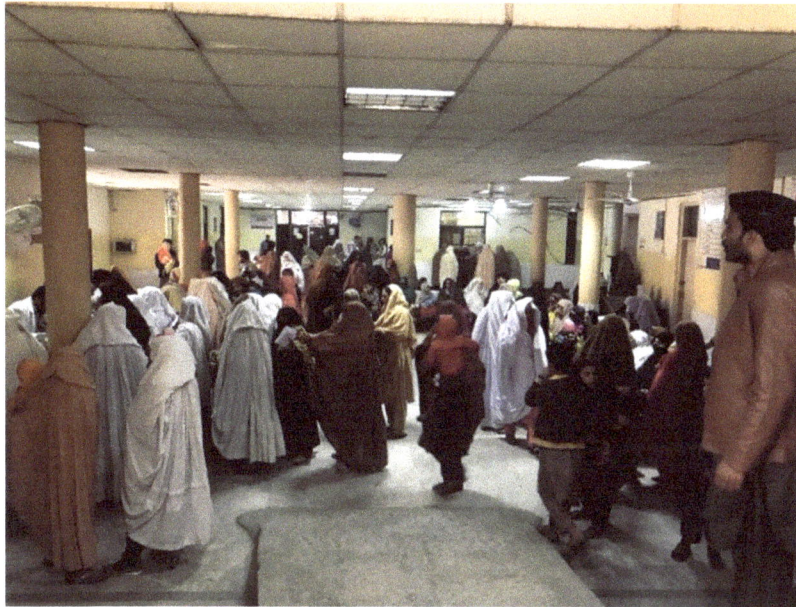

Overcrowded hospital. Patients, mostly women and children, fill the outpatient department reception at the Moulvi Ameer Shah Qadri Memorial Hospital in Peshawar (photo by Michael Niechzial).

2035. Like admitted hospital care, projected demand for outpatient care for Khyber Pakhtunkhwa is adjusted for demand-side factors as determined by the difference in service provision and capacity for the baseline year of 2015, which results in the requirement of 105.4 million outpatient consultations projected for the province in 2020, growing to 223.2 million by 2035 at an average annual growth rate of 7.4%. The assumption of outpatient facilities being open 6 days a week, standard consultation times, and an occupancy of 85% translates to a demand of 15,879 outpatient consultation rooms across public and private sectors and hospital and clinic settings in 2020, growing to 34,440 rooms by 2035 (see Appendix 4 for the methodology used for modeling demand for health care).[35]

Inappropriate infrastructure (buildings and installations). The infrastructure was inappropriate in almost all facilities visited. It included often outdated facilities in terms of (i) standard requirements for adequate spaces (consultation rooms with less than 16 square meters and 2–3 doctors and patients inside, no equipment for clinical examination let alone of privacy); (ii) issues related to infection control (e.g., a tuberculosis lab at the dead-end of a corridor); (iii) long distances between services that should be interlinked and close to each other (e.g., ICU and operational therapy areas); (iv) basic installations for utilities (power and water supply, sanitary installations, and sewage system); (v) solid waste management (incinerators are absent or not functional) partially due to the lack of preventive and curative maintenance; and (vi) hospitals being either too big (one THQ hospital with 150 beds) or too small for the number of patients they receive, specifically in the outpatient departments (OPDs).

---

[35] F. Ng. 2018. *Khyber Pakhtunkhwa Planning for Physical and Human Resources.* Background paper for the Assessment of the Khyber Pakhtunkhwa Health Sector. Peshawar. 13–15 February.

Two hospitals that the team visited have been totally or partially accommodated in buildings that have never been planned and constructed for this purpose, posing serious problems with regard to patient and staff safety (hygiene or infection prevention) and the organization (efficiency) of workflows.[36]

The box below refers to the standards for the ICU location in a hospital as established by the health building notes of the United Kingdom's National Health Service. Similar standards exist for patient wards and other functional areas of the hospital.

Box: Standards for Intensive Care Unit Adjacencies: Health Building Notes of the United Kingdom's National Health Service

For clinical reasons, the intensive care unit (ICU) should be easily accessible to the areas to which patients are usually admitted, such as the accident and emergency department, recovery room, surgical and medical wards. Health building note 27 suggests that the ICU should be near the theaters to enable engineering services to be shared, but this is by no means an overriding factor: a separation of engineering plant may increase failure protection.

An easy access to high dependency units results in significant advantages in case of patient evacuation in the event of fire or decanting in the event of closure, and for both units as a step-down or step-up facility.

Increasingly, it is desirable to site the ICU close to the imaging department. Since there exist near-patient laboratory facilities, this makes access to main pathology laboratories less important.

A meticulous mapping of department can aid in optimizing the distance patients are moved. In addition, in locations with heavy flow of patients, wider corridors and large lifts are required.

Optimizing the location of the ICU relative to ambulance access is essential for facilities that are prone to receiving transfers from outside hospitals.

Patients receiving coronary care and routine post-operative care (recovery) should have a separate area or ward, although they may share facilities and staff.

Source: Index of Design and Construction http://www.icdkwt.com/pdf/policiesandguidelines/ DesignandConstruction/ Guidelines for Intensive Care Units Design-2008.pdf. p.5.

---

[36] The Moulvi Ameer Shah Qadri Memorial (Women and Children) Hospital was initially built as a logistics office and workshop for public bus services, and then modified to accommodate outpatient services for approximately 200,000 patient contacts per annum in 2017 and inpatient admissions of around 8,500 patients with an average length of stay (ALOS) of 4.9 days accommodated in 131 beds corresponding to a bed occupancy rate of approximately 87%. A new building of 108 beds is only partially occupied (including a cardiac care unit established on a personal initiative of one medical doctor). The Naseer Ullah Khan Babar Memorial, a provincial referral hospital by category, was initially constructed as a medical supplies department store, and then transformed because of need (catchment population of around 1 million)—OPD's 2,500–3,000 patients per day, A&E cases of more than 1,000 per day, no ICU, no blood bank, no waste disposal system, no space for extension and low bed occupancy.

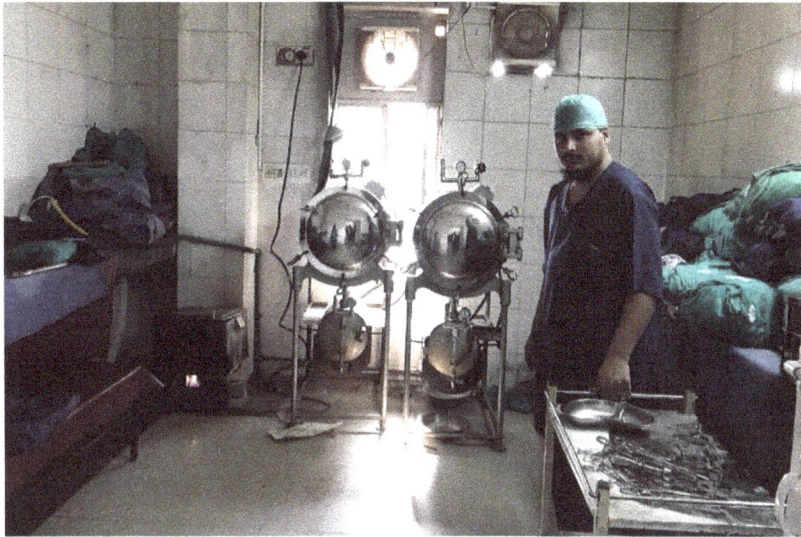

Outdated equipment and inadequate workflow. A medical doctor shows the small central sterile supply department of the Naseer Ullah Khan Babar Memorial Hospital in Peshawar with old and obsolete medical equipment, which affect the working process (photo by Michael Niechzial).

The same principle is valid for medical equipment, from basic diagnostic equipment required for medical consultation to more sophisticated imaging, laboratory, sterilization, occupational therapy and ICU, and anesthesia machines.

According to the Service Delivery Indicators Survey conducted by a team of the Khyber Medial University (KMU), all of the visited hospitals had weighing scales, stethoscopes, and sphygmomanometers (for blood pressure measurement), but only one (Emergency Satellite Hospital Nowshera) had a functioning computed topography (CT) scanner and magnetic resonance imaging (MRI) machine made available to the hospital in the framework of a PPP arrangement, and no mammography machine was available in any of the visited hospitals. Specifically at OPDs, even though provided by clinical specialists, only PHC services (auscultation, prescription) are being offered to most of the patients. As a consequence, many of the secondary level hospitals function as large outpatient clinics with patient turnovers, suggesting both a high percentage of PHC cases as well as the rather limited quality of care.

Limited time for consultations and examinations and unbalanced load of inpatient services. According to the data collected by the KMU team (Table 6) only 3.5–10.0 minutes is available for consultation, examination, and providing advice to patients and/or their parents and relatives—and this is based on the rather ideal assumption that OPD visits would be equally spread over the time of each working day (8 hours or 480 minutes). In reality, however, consultation hours are usually between 8 a.m. and 12 noon or 1 p.m. at the latest, i.e., the time effectively available is limited to 4–5 hours only, and average consultation time is significantly short. This pattern is also confirmed by the high number of patient contacts in the accident and emergency (A&E) unit. Most of these visits are not related to real accidents or medical emergencies but visits occurring outside of the usual consultation hours. The rather short average length of stay (ALOS) (2.0–3.6 days) of all cases admitted for inpatient care also indicates a rather low share of severely

Table 6: Performance Data of the Most Frequented Secondary Level Hospitals, 2017

	Name	OPD Visits	A&E visits	Visits / Day	Consult Rooms	Consults / Room / Day	Average Consult Time (min)	Inpatient Beds	Patients Admitted	% of OPD Visits	ALOS	Inpatient Days	BOR
1	DHQ Abbottabad	380,283	176,526	2.27	22	103	4:65	370	62,276	11	3	186,828	138
2	DHQ Dir Upper	225,500	7,576	951	20	48	10:09	230	26,272	11	2	52,544	63
3	DHQ Haripur	374,267	204,613	2.36	20	118	4:06	210	27,483	5	3	82,449	108
4	NUBH, Peshawar	352,173	309,724	2.70	25	108	4:44	119	15,374	2	3,6	55,346	127
5	ESH Nowshera	169,023	66,990	963	10	96	4:98	70	4,606	2	2	9,212	36
6	DHQ Swabi	226,143	104,983	1.35	10	135	3:55	60	13,737	4	2	27,474	125
7	DHQ Shangla	123,249	19,632	583	9	65	7:41	60	6,986	5	4	27,944	128

A&E = accident and emergency, ALOS = average length of stay, BOR = bed occupancy rate, DHQ = district headquarters, ESH = Emergency Satellite Hospital, NUBH = Naseer Uddin Babar Hospital, OPD = outpatient department.

Source: Data from the Khyber Medical University. 2017. Service Delivery Indicator Survey. Peshawar.

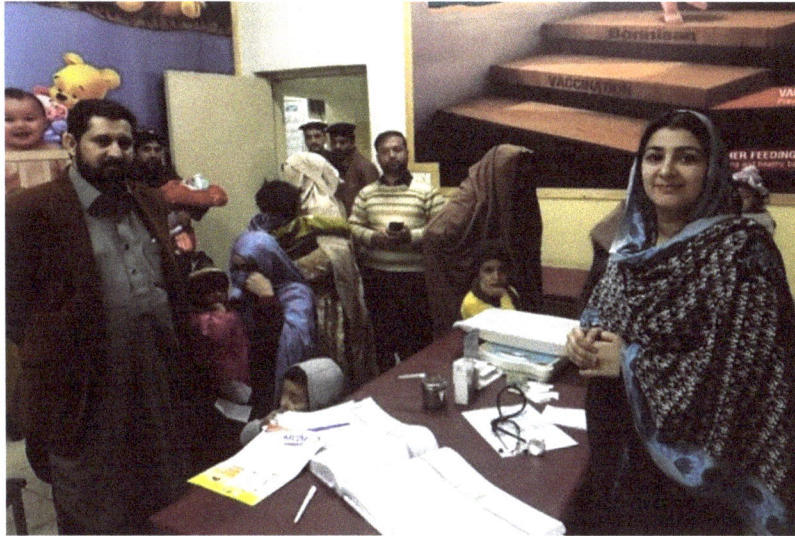

Pediatric specialty consultation. Two doctors and several patients crowd into one consultation room with no equipment and with long waiting line at the Moulvi Ameer Shah Qadri Memorial Hospital, Peshawar (photo by Michael Niechzial).

ill patients with advanced stages of their disease, a low prevalence of multi-morbidity in the hospitalized patients, and a limited number of people at advanced age or patients with other risk factors leading to higher frequency of clinical complications and consequently a longer duration of their stay at the hospital.

At the Abbottabad and Dir Upper DHQ hospitals the share of patients undergoing any kind of minor or major surgical intervention is below 10% (9.87% minor and 3.71% major). At the Haripur and Shangla DHQ hospitals the rate is at 13.03% and 14.43%, respectively. Only at the Swabi DHQ hospital and the Naseer Uddin Babar Hospital in Peshawar are rates of 22.14% and 22.97% reached levels expected from a secondary level referral hospital. Exceptionally high is the rate at the Emergency Satellite Hospital Nowshera (46.29%) showing it fulfills its specialized referral function.

Inpatient care is indirectly suffering from overload at the OPDs. Except for the Emergency Satellite Hospital Nowshera and the DHQ Dir Upper, bed occupancy rates are above 100%, indicating an extremely high turnover rate (two patients in one bed on the same day) confirmed by a correspondingly low ALOS (Table 6). A low ALOS is not a negative outcome, however, considering the relatively low number of surgeries in most of the facilities and the low number of deliveries or days in many of them (despite the still high maternal mortality rate in the province), it can be stated that the DHQ and other referral level hospitals do not fulfill their referral function.

Limited understanding of renal dialysis services and capacity. Renal dialysis services and capacity in Khyber Pakhtunkhwa are not well known despite the increasing prevalence of end-stage renal failure over the years. Hospital and center-based hemodialysis for renal failure is modeled separately from acute overnight care, as it is provided on a same-day basis in stabilized patients. Dialysis options are broadly categorized into hemodialysis and peritoneal dialysis, with either type provided in-home or hospital and/or center-based. The reference countries used to inform the modeling provide in-home and hospital and/or center-based dialysis on a 1:1 basis,

Table 7: Inpatient Services at Surveyed Hospitals

Name	DHQ Abbottabad	DHQ Dir Upper	DHQ Haripur	NUBH, Peshawar	ESH Nowshera	DHQ Swabi	DHQ Shangla
Surgeries / work day (no.)	22.57	3.59	14.57	12.97	7.83	11.17	3.34
Surgeries / day / OT (no.)	7.52	0.72	2.43	2.16	3.92	2.79	3.34
Deliveries (no.)	21,667	2,503	6,725	4,190	1,855	4,354	1,366
Deliveries / day (no.)	59	7	18	11	5	12	4

ALOS = average length of stay, BOR = bed occupancy rate, DHQ = district headquarters, ESH = Emergency Satellite Hospital, NUBH = Naseer Uddin Babar Hospital, OT = overtime.

Source: Data from the Khyber Medical University. 2017. *Service Delivery Indicator Survey*. Peshawar.

i.e., 50% of patients require facility-based dialysis. The modeling hospital and center-based dialysis projects that demand will increase rapidly from patients requiring facility-based dialysis, from 2,580 in 2020 to over 5,800 patients in 2035, as a result of the high burden of disease, risk factors, and population aging in the province, and of the improvements in access to chronic dialysis services over time. Conversion to dialysis machines is based on the current practice of twice-weekly dialysis, with a gradually increasing frequency toward the internationally-accepted and evidence-based frequency of three times a week per patient. Assuming machines will be operated 6 days a week with a throughput of 2.5 dialysis patients per day, 344 hemodialysis machines are required in hospitals and centers across Khyber Pakhtunkhwa, increasing to 1,006 by 2035 (Table 8).

Table 8: Projected Demand for Episodes and Capacity for Dialysis, 2020–2035

	2020	2025	2030	2035
Hospital/center-based dialysis patients	268,298	389,094	558,100	784,291
Weekly frequency	2.00	2.2	2.4	2.6
Episodes	2,580	3,401	4,472	5,801
Dialysis machines	344	499	716	1,006

Source: Government of Khyber Pakhtunkhwa, Department of Health. 2017.

Health workforce shortage. A pillar of the health system is its workforce, and in Khyber Pakhtunkhwa, modeled projections for medical practitioners by specialties indicate that more than 15,500 full-time equivalent doctors are required to deliver services to the population in 2020, growing to over 56,000 by 2035. The greatest increases required by specialty in medical practitioners are for vascular surgery, medical oncology, nephrology, ENT surgery, geriatric medicine, emergency medicine, hematology, and urology, all with average annual growth rates greater than 20%. The medical workforce is supported by nurses and midwives, with projections that 46,000 full-time equivalent nurses—made up of support nurses, registered nurses, and midwives—are required to deliver services to Pakistan's population in 2020, growing to over 176,000 nurses required by 2035. Unfortunately, doctors are not adequately supported by a qualified nursing workforce. More needs to be done to secure adequate support of these doctors by qualified nurses, midwives, and other medico-technical staff. With all planned positions filled, the doctor-to-nurse (including midwives) ratio would be 1:3, whereas a ratio of 1:4 and above is recommended (although Pakistan is not the only country with a bias toward medical doctors in the composition of their health workforce).[37] Table 9 shows the plan and filled health workforce in 2018 that clearly confirms the inadequate number of qualified staff. Recruiting qualified nurses in sufficient numbers is a key challenge when striving for better quality of hospital care. Where there seems to be a lack of qualified staff, there is a plethora of non-health workers representing more than a third of the total workforce in almost all surveyed hospitals, leading to high (above 2.5) staff-to-bed ratios (Table 10). Following international benchmarks, an efficiently organized district hospital would have a staff-to-bed ratio of not more than 2.

Table 9: Planned and Filled Health Workforce, 2018

	Staff Positions Filled of Specialists			Staff Positions Filled of General Practitioners			Staff Positions Filled of Paramedical Staff			Staff Positions Filled: All Categories		
	Plan	Filled	% Filled	Plan	Filled	% Filled	Plan	Filled	% Filled	Plan	Filled	% Filled
Total	437	247	57	2,306	1,652	72	7,945	7,193	91	10,688	9,092	85

Source: Department of Health (District Health Information System). 2018.

Lack of quality assurance mechanisms. None of the visited hospitals have quality assurance mechanisms. The team could not find any of the following: (i) written standard clinical protocols and pathways for diagnostic and therapeutic procedures; (ii) established or operational quality circles or committees; or (iii) monitoring, feedback, or review mechanisms for key performance and quality indicators. This is despite the fact that many of the staff interviewed confirmed the necessity of such tools and instruments of process management to guarantee minimum quality levels of care.

---

[37] WHO. 2006. Chapter 1: Health Workers: A Global Profile. In *Working Together for Health: The World Health Report 2006.* Geneva.

Table 10: Health Workforce Composition at Surveyed Hospitals

Name	DHQ Abbottabad	DHQ Dir Upper	DHQ Haripur	NUBH, Peshawar	ESH Nowshera	DHQ Swabi	DHQ A. Shangla
Health workers (no.)	593	197	231	263	150	140	185
Registered nurses (no.)	125	54	129	67	40	51	48
Medical staff (no.)	115	7	67	103	51	18	46
Non-health workers (no.)	313	314	134	126	147	72	69
Total Staff	**906**	**511**	**365**	**389**	**297**	**212**	**254**
Non-health workers (% of total)	34.55	61.45	36.71	32.39	49.49	33.96	27.17
Staff / hospital bed	2.45	2.22	1.74	3.27	4.24	3.53	4.23

DHQ = district headquarters, ESH = Emergency Satellite Hospital, NUBH = Naseer Uddin Babar Hospital.

Note: Total staff = health workers + non-health workers.

Source: Data from the Khyber Medical University. 2017. Service Delivery Indicator Survey. Peshawar.

Limited drug supplies. Only essential drugs provided through the medical supply department are available at the hospital, and even for those, frequent stockouts have been reported. Hospitals working as referral centers should have the opportunity to procure the drugs and consumables they need, based on principles of clinical evidence for medical treatment, rational use of resources through preference given to generic drugs, and compliance with quality control procedures assuring that the product does not harm and contains the elements listed on the drug package or container.

Limited monitoring and evaluation. No analysis of data and indicators has been undertaken in any of the visited hospitals to evaluate the outcomes of clinical care, at least in terms of inpatient morbidity and mortality that may be directly or indirectly related to the medical intervention (e.g., hospital-acquired infection). However, the DOH website does display infection protocols, which means these protocols are available but yet to be notified for implementation. The maternal mortality rates are still high in Khyber Pakhtunkhwa,[38] but no mortality audit has taken place (neither in the hospitals visited nor elsewhere).

V.   Recommendations

Given current shortages in capacity and human resources modeled from international benchmarks at a population-based level and adjusted for local circumstances in Khyber Pakhtunkhwa, it is judicious that the DOH initiate and implement a development program that responds to the growing and changing health needs of the population in locations with the greatest relative need. This goal requires greater capacity tracking and reporting for both public and private health care facilities to be able to determine district capacity accurately. Mechanisms to facilitate this goal are already in place with the independent monitoring unit (IMU) and Health Care Commission (HCC), both of which can provide access and information collection of physical and human resources for planning purposes.

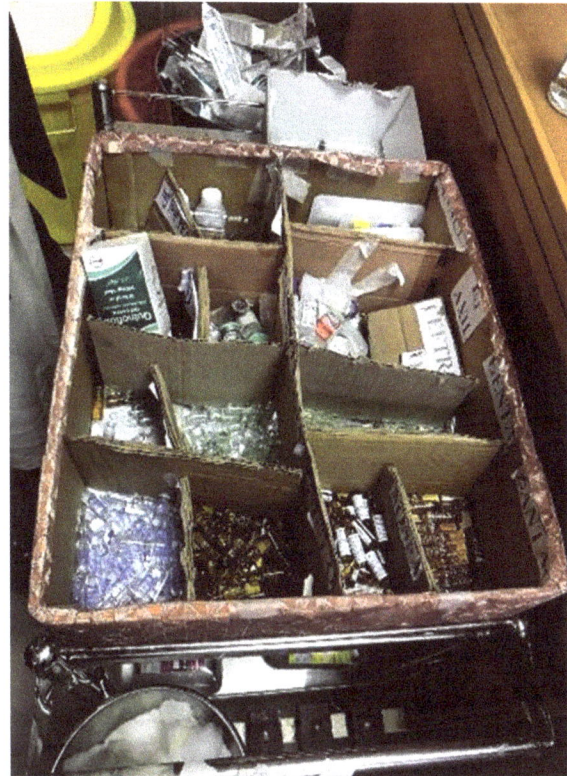

Limited drug supplies. The risk of emergency drugs running out of stock is high at the accident and emergency unit of the Qazi Hussain Ahmad Medical Complex, Nowshera (photo by Michael Niechzial).

Notwithstanding these limitations in the geographic location of new developments, the following are recommended:

Facility Capacity and Human Resources Improvements

1. Development of hospital bed capacity in Charsadda, Dera Ismail Khan, Kohistan, Mansehra, Mardan, Nowshera, Swab, and Swat districts of category A and B hospitals should be prioritized.
2. The DOH should embark on a program to deliver two category A hospitals, three category B hospitals, seven category C hospitals or an alternative combination to provide 700–900 public hospital beds annually across Khyber Pakhtunkhwa.

---

[38] According to the Khyber Pakhtunkhwa DHIS Annual Report 2017, the maternal mortality (ratio) was 183/100,000 live births—the actual (absolute) number of women who died after birth in one of the public health care facilities reporting to the DHIS (district headquarter hospitals = 83% of all registered deliveries, *tehsil* headquarter hospitals = 13%, and rural health centers = 3%, basic health units = 1%) was 395 (the total number of live births registered was 215,514). It shall be noted that this figure does not include deliveries managed in private facilities and in tertiary-level care facilities, and consequently the ratio (and number) may be biased in two ways: Higher than real average as private facilities tend to transfer cases at risk to public facilities; lower than average because complicated cases managed in tertiary care hospitals are not taken into consideration. The total estimated number of deliveries in the Khyber Pakhtunkhwa Province in 2017 was approximately 400,000. Data from Ministry of Health, Directorate General Health Services, Khyber Pakhtunkhwa, Peshawar: District Health Information System (DHIS)—Annual Report 2017 (www.dhiskp.gov.pk/reports/Annual%20 Report%202017%20N.pdf.

3. An upfront investment in upscaling dialysis services across hospitals should be made, with the existing renal dialysis unit.
4. The DOH should embark on a program to deliver an additional 30–40 dialysis machines across hospital facilities each year.
5. Tertiary education facilities (both public and private) should be equipped to educate and train a minimum of 2,000 medical graduates and 5,000 nursing personnel and equivalent.

Quality Care and Quality Management Improvements

Building on recent initiatives by the Government of Khyber Pakhtunkhwa to strengthen quality management in the health care system in general and in hospitals in particular (e.g., the establishment of HCC), a systematic approach should be followed to improve quality of care. This approach would include measures to introduce and strengthen compliance with standard operating procedures (SOPs) (clinical guidelines and pathways) to reduce arbitrary variations in diagnostic and therapeutic procedures leading to ineffective and inefficient provision of care. In cooperation with the Pakistan National Accreditation Council, norms and standards for secondary level hospitals[39] can be adapted (harmonized with national standards) and a provincial accreditation system can be developed (to be managed by the HCC) and introduced as a basic measure to assure minimum quality standards (at least with regard to structural or input factors such as infrastructure, equipment, and staffing). Three core elements of quality management need to be developed and systematically introduced into the province's health care system:

1. **Standard operating procedures.** With a few exceptions, no SOPs like guidelines and clinical pathways exist or are in use in hospital-based inpatient and outpatient care. Although this does not mean that diagnosis and treatment are made without any reference, as guidance is being provided and control is being assured by heads of departments or senior (specialist) doctors. This implies, however, that clinical case is managed on a hierarchical model of organization, rather than a modern, interdisciplinary, interprofessional, team-oriented, and transparent model that is based on predefined standards following international best practice and considering scientific evidence. What is further needed is the elaboration of clinical guidelines and protocols for the most frequent diseases and medical conditions that would require admission to secondary level inpatient care. The target is around 85% of the volume of services provided at the secondary level. Usually the 10 most frequent diseases and conditions of all four basic disciplines—internal medicine, pediatrics, surgery, and gynecology or obstetrics—are sufficient to reach this target. See Figure 6 below for good practice examples of SOPs for medical care.

2. **Framework for continuous quality improvement.** Currently, no framework exists to promote quality of care at secondary hospitals in Khyber Pakhtunkhwa. The abovementioned protocols would only be one element. Two pillars need to be built to create a comprehensive framework for continuous quality improvement (CQI), which is the ultimate objective of quality management in any sector not only at service or facility level but also at the level of the (provincial) health care system—(i) internal quality management (including clinical protocols and pathways), and (ii) external quality management (benchmarking with hospitals of the same level). Results achieved with internal quality management measures—indicator monitoring and the establishment

---

[39] See standards developed with support provided by the Deutsche Gesellschaft für Internationale Zusammenarbeit and I. Thaver and M. Khalid. 2016. *Final Report: Secondary Level Minimum Health Services Delivery Package for Secondary Care Hospitals (MHSDP)*.

Figure 6: Good Example of Quality Improvement Tools and Mechanisms (Guidelines/Clinical Pathways) for Patients with Symptoms of Heart Failure

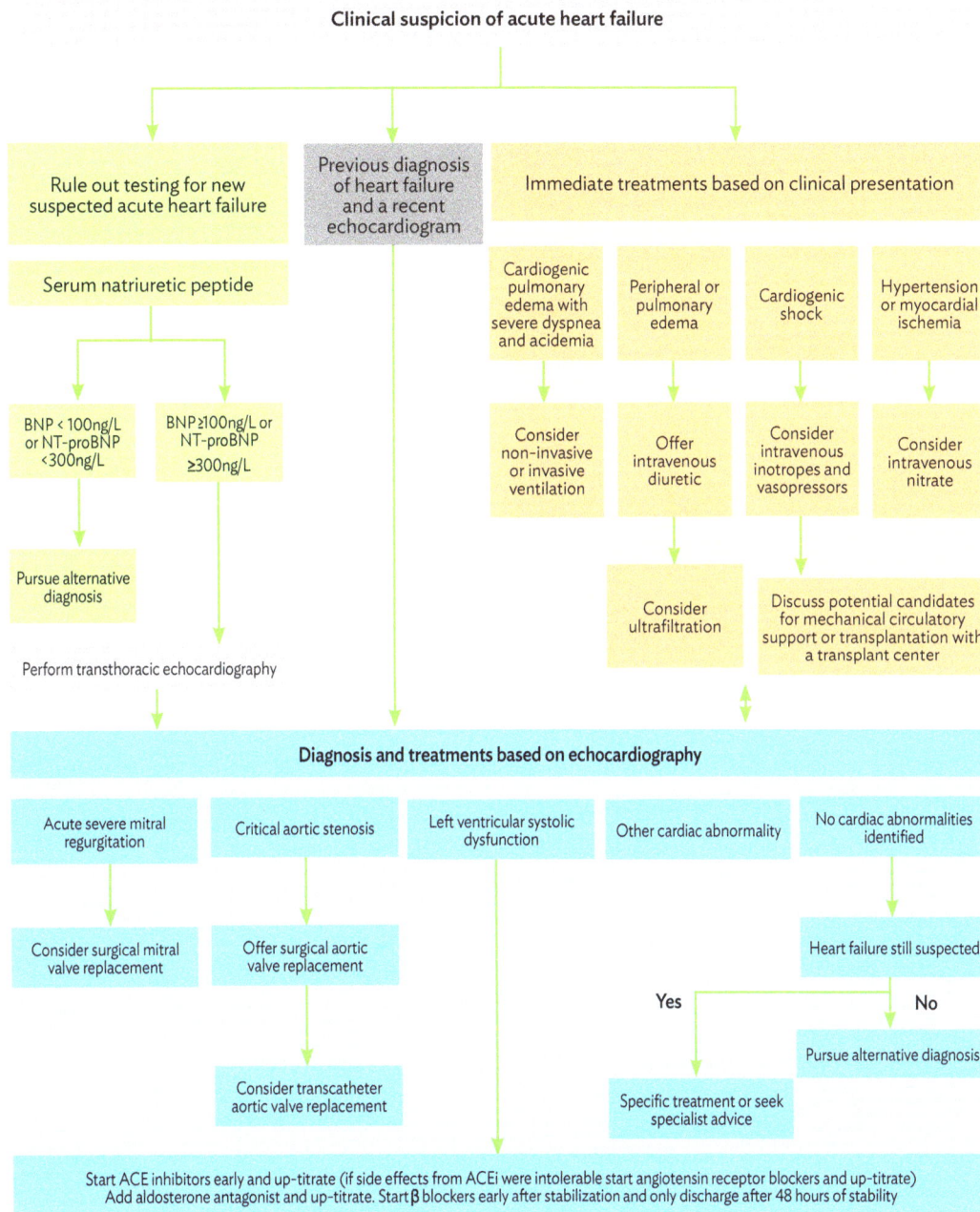

Clinical suspicion of acute heart failure

Rule out testing for new suspected acute heart failure

Previous diagnosis of heart failure and a recent echocardiogram

Immediate treatments based on clinical presentation

Serum natriuretic peptide

BNP < 100ng/L or NT-proBNP <300ng/L

BNP ≥100ng/L or NT-proBNP ≥300ng/L

Pursue alternative diagnosis

Perform transthoracic echocardiography

Cardiogenic pulmonary edema with severe dyspnea and acidemia

Peripheral or pulmonary edema

Cardiogenic shock

Hypertension or myocardial ischemia

Consider non-invasive or invasive ventilation

Offer intravenous diuretic

Consider intravenous inotropes and vasopressors

Consider intravenous nitrate

Consider ultrafiltration

Discuss potential candidates for mechanical circulatory support or transplantation with a transplant center

Diagnosis and treatments based on echocardiography

Acute severe mitral regurgitation

Critical aortic stenosis

Left ventricular systolic dysfunction

Other cardiac abnormality

No cardiac abnormalities identified

Consider surgical mitral valve replacement

Offer surgical aortic valve replacement

Heart failure still suspected

Yes   No

Pursue alternative diagnosis

Consider transcatheter aortic valve replacement

Specific treatment or seek specialist advice

Start ACE inhibitors early and up-titrate (if side effects from ACEi were intolerable start angiotensin receptor blockers and up-titrate) Add aldosterone antagonist and up-titrate. Start β blockers early after stabilization and only discharge after 48 hours of stability

ACE = angiotensin-converting enzyme, BNP = brain natriuretic peptide, NT-proBNP = N-terminal pro brain natriuretic peptide.

Source: K. Dworzynski et al. 2014. Diagnosing and Managing Acute Heart Failure in Adults: Summary of NICE Guidance. *The BMJ*. 349 (g5695). October. doi: 10.1136/bmj.g5695.

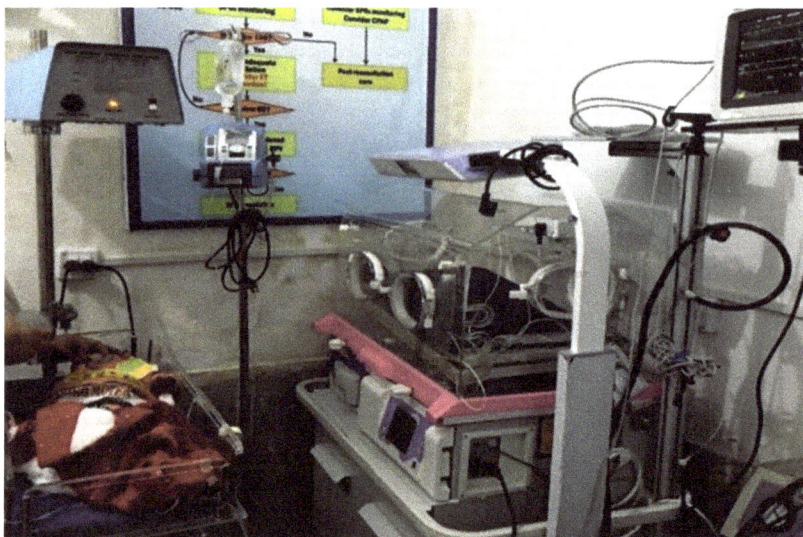

Good practice example. Guideline for the resuscitation of newborns is fixed on the wall of the neonatology unit at the Swabi DHQ Hospital (photo by Michael Niechzial).

of quality circles or committees including mortality conferences analyzing quality issues and discussing, implementing, or monitoring the implementation of corrective measures—shall be documented in annual quality reports to be established by all (public and private) facilities offering secondary level care. The availability of such reports could become a licensing or accreditation criterion. With regard to external quality management, the DOH (quality department) shall collect data from all hospitals on selected indicators and analyze those data by comparing the results and their core services against each other. This process will need to take into consideration the patient mix the hospitals are dealing with to avoid bias in the evaluation due to "cream skimming" by health care providers (e.g., through early transfer to tertiary-level hospitals) and other measures to purposely or unintentionally manipulate data on clinical outcomes. This kind of benchmarking will help both health care facility managers and the DOH to monitor and improve the quality of care (see Appendix 4 for a detailed description and examples).

3. **Continuous medical education.** The protocols and pathways and the systematic quality management processes and related tools and instruments at health care facilities require regular updating of knowledge and skills of all medical, paramedical, technical, and administrative staff through training and other capacity-building measures (e.g., e-learning courses, on-site coaching or mentoring, peer review of medical records and clinical practice, staff exchange programs, certified training offered by national and international third-party providers, etc.). Participation in such measures and events should be mandatory for all staff and documented and monitored through a credit points account (see Appendix 4 for a detailed description and examples).

CHAPTER 4
Health Financing

I.   Overview

This chapter presents an overview and analysis of health financing in Khyber Pakhtunkhwa with (i) the current status and challenges shown according to the health financing functions of revenue collection, pooling, and purchasing; and (ii) the issues in the health insurance program the province introduced 2 years ago as part of its pursuit of universal health coverage (UHC). The chapter also examines the current state of public financial management (PFM) in the health sector given the key role that appropriate PFM mechanisms play in ensuring sustainable financing for UHC. The PFM challenges are also presented in each of the health financing functions using the WHO framework in aligning PFM and health financing (footnote 16). The section ends with recommendations on health financing actions that can help move forward UHC.

II.   Achievements

Establishment of the Sehat Sahulat Program. The Government of Khyber Pakhtunkhwa launched the SHPI (Sehat Sahulat Program) in 2015 in four districts with the financial support of the German government through KfW. Utilizing its own financial resources, the provincial government had scaled up the SHPI to cover an estimated 69% of the province's poorest population. It is mobilizing PRs3.8 billion ($32.9 million) annually to cover administrative costs and fully subsidize the premium of 2,488,000 households (approximately 19,990,000 individuals). The SHPI pays for inpatient secondary and tertiary health care services. The cost of the program includes premium and administrative expenses, which are provided through the State Life Insurance Corporation of Pakistan (SLIC) by the completion of its third phase. The establishment of the SHPI, along with the progressive increase in the percentage of the population covered by SHPI, was a major step toward achieving UHC in the province. The SHPI is managed through the SLIC, which was selected after national competitive bidding. With the launch and expansion of the SHPI, a larger purchaser is being established and a purchaser-provider split has been inherently built into its design; both public and private providers are being enrolled into the program through contracts. As a province-wide single government health insurance program, SHPI can leverage its purchasing power to promote health interventions that best benefit the health of the general population.

Improvement in public financial management. Implementation of the SHPI and other UHC-related reforms in Khyber Pakhtunkhwa needs a sound PFM system. Fortunately, the province is moving in this direction as shown by improvements in the 2017 PFM assessment compared with the 2007 PFM assessment. Based on these two assessments, budget credibility improved with the variance between budgeted and actual expenditures decreasing over 10 years both at the aggregate level and by composition. The overall budgeting process remained well organized and participatory with extensive guidance to line departments and with general adherence to budget calendar by line departments. The multiyear perspective in fiscal planning, expenditure policy, and budgeting advanced with the approval and implementation of the Khyber Pakhtunkhwa Integrated Development Strategy. Public access to key fiscal information improved with the release of in-year budget execution reports. The promulgation of Khyber Pakhtunkhwa Public Procurement Regulatory Authority Act, 2012 and Khyber Pakhtunkhwa Public Procurement Regulatory Authority Rules 2014 yielded improvements in the procurement regime, including (i) enhanced procurement monitoring, (ii) upgraded public access to procurement information, and (iii) comprehensive procurement compliant management system. The rollout of the government financial management information system has also enhanced the quality of information in the budget execution reports.

III.   Current Status and Challenges

Revenue Collection

The Khyber Pakhtunkhwa health system is financed by government revenues, private funds, and external sources from developing partners. In FY2016, private out-of-pocket (OOP) payments accounted for the largest share of total health expenditures at 72.4%, with government revenues at 16.4% and contributions by official donor agencies at 0.9% (Appendix 6).

Federal transfers, which are sourced mostly from general taxes from income and sales, constitute the main source of government revenue funding in the Government of Khyber Pakhtunkhwa, as they make up nearly two-thirds of total budgeted revenue in FY2018.[40] Other relevant sources of income include foreign loans (about 9% of total), foreign grants (about 5%), provincial tax receipts (about 4%), and profits from hydroelectricity (about 3%).

The provincial finance department then provides (i) the financing to the provincial government, including for the delivery of health services by province-managed health care providers; and (ii) funds to the district governments, which are then obliged to spend the money on health for their constituencies (Figure 7).

As mentioned, the Government of Khyber Pakhtunkhwa is also paying premiums for the SHPI. Apart from the SHPI, other mechanisms for paying for health are those in autonomous government bodies or corporations under the federal and provincial governments, wherein they independently finance their health facilities and reimburse health care expenses of their employees. Financing by private funds mainly comprises employers' funds and households' OOP expenses on health care, with OOP expenses accounting for nearly three-fourths of total health spending, as discussed previously. **This high share of OOP cost indicates a regressive funding mechanism**, which contributes to deterring access to needed health care services.

---

[40] Government of Khyber Pakhtunkhwa, Department of Finance. 2017.

Figure 7: Flow of Government Funds to Health Facilities

```
                    Department of Finance
        Budget transfer              One line item transfer

    KP–Provincial health              District governments
        department
                         Budget transfer        Budget transfer
        Budget transfer
                         District health          Other
                             setup                sector

                         Budget transfer

  Public health facilities    Public health facilities
  managed by the provincial   managed by the district
  health department-          governments–including
  including DHQH              THQH
```

DHQH = district headquarters hospital, THQH = *tehsil* headquarters hospital.

Source: Author's diagram based on Government of Khyber Pakhtunkhwa, Department of Finance. 2017.

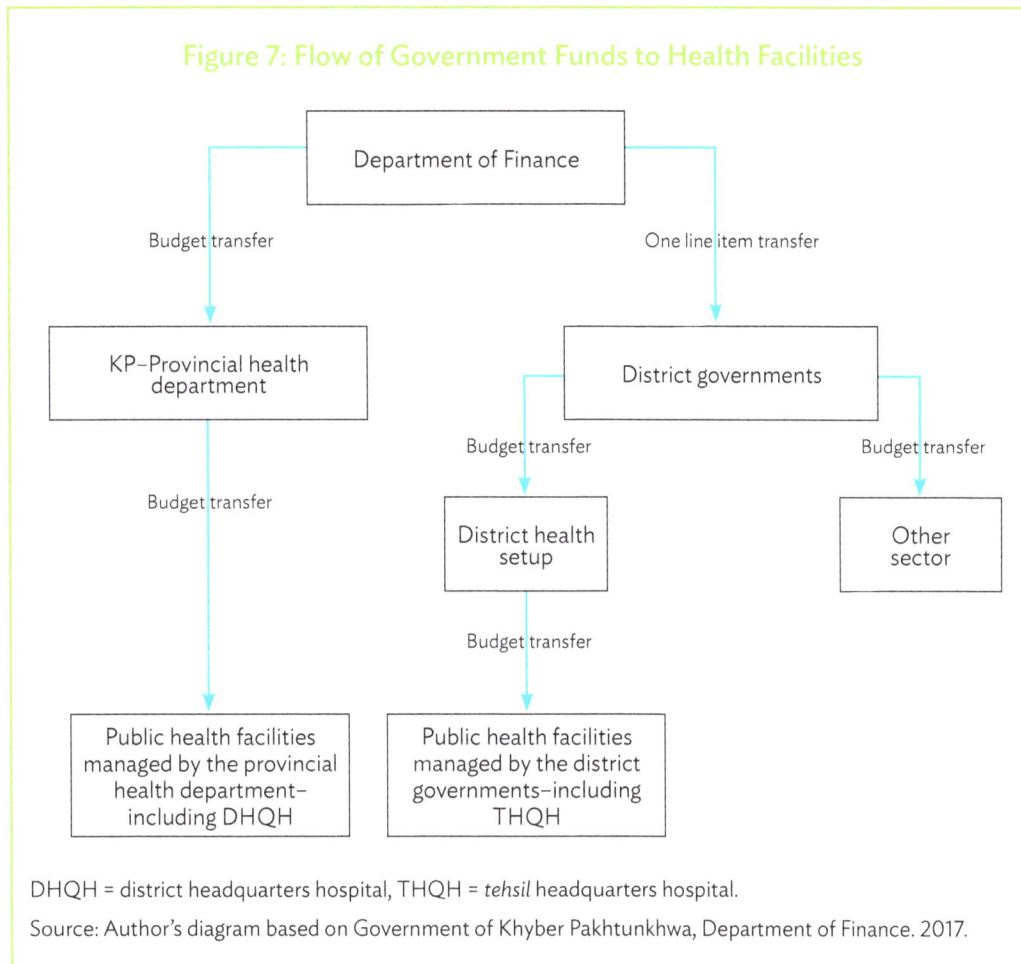

Fiscal space for health can be expanded (to increase funding for health care) through increased government revenue.[41] Enhanced fiscal space can be achieved through increased general tax revenues, other than economic growth. Pakistan has a low tax-to-GDP ratio—12.6%[42] in 2016. Although this is an increase from the 2015 tax-to-GDP ratio of 11.0%, the International Monetary Fund notes that Pakistan could nearly double its tax revenues to 22.3% of its GDP,[43] thus showing that there is a room for increasing funding for health in Pakistan, and by extension for Khyber Pakhtunkhwa. The recent announcement by the Ministry of National Health Services, Regulations and Coordination (NHSRC) about introducing a sin tax on cigarettes and sugary beverages and its utilization for health sector funding is a step in the right direction; however, the exact amount of tax to be imposed and the distribution of sin tax among health sector programs and provinces are not yet clear.

[41] WHO. Health Financing for Universal Coverage. http://www.who.int/health_financing/topics/fiscal-space/main-drivers/en/.

[42] ADB. 2017. *Key Indicators for Asia and the Pacific 2017*. Manila. https://www.adb.org/publications/key-indicators-asia-and-pacific-2017.

[43] S. Cevik. 2016. Unlocking Pakistan's Revenue Potential. *IMF Working Paper*. No. 16/182. Washington, DC: International Monetary Fund.

The ongoing reforms in tax administration in the province by the Khyber Pakhtunkhwa Revenue Authority, established in 2013 to collect sales tax on services, have helped increase tax revenues. Currently, the sales tax on services has become the largest source of provincial taxes at 58%. However, more improvements can be made as the DOH is still developing systems and capacity for revenue-compliance risk management, and institutional mechanisms for fiscal reporting have yet to improve in capturing the extra-budgetary operations and information on off-budget donor-funded projects, which remain outside the overall budgetary figures for the province. **Significant improvements in tax administration performance (particularly in the areas of transparency of taxpayer obligations and liabilities) and in registration, assessment, and collection of taxes** are still needed.

Pooling

Of the funds that are pooled in Khyber Pakhtunkhwa, government revenue is the largest pool of health financing. Table 11 shows the consolidated current budget of the health sector from 2012 to 2018, which indicates an increasing trend. This pool has increased in recent years, as shown by the increasing sectoral share of the health sector in the province[44] from 6.7% in FY2013 to 11% in FY2018 (Figure 8).

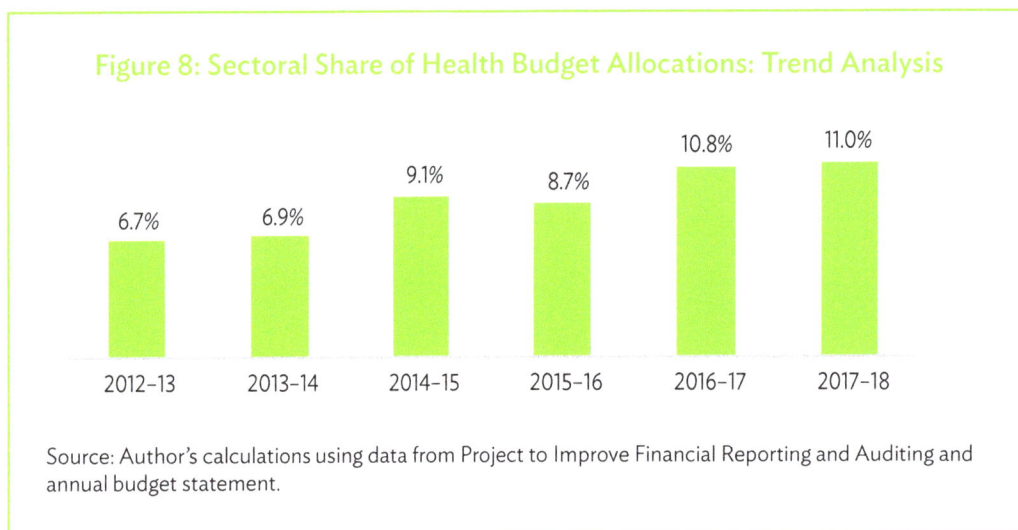

Figure 8: Sectoral Share of Health Budget Allocations: Trend Analysis

6.7%	6.9%	9.1%	8.7%	10.8%	11.0%
2012–13	2013–14	2014–15	2015–16	2016–17	2017–18

Source: Author's calculations using data from Project to Improve Financial Reporting and Auditing and annual budget statement.

Table 11: Consolidated Current Budget of Health Sector
(PRs million)

Budget by Funding Stream	2012–2013	2013–2014	2014–2015	2015–2016	2016–2017	2017–2018
Current budget	20,449	31,226	34,230	30,937	45,523	49,280
Development budget	9,965	10,762	15,662	13,458	15,662	17,190
Total	**30,414**	**41,988**	**49,892**	**44,395**	**61,185**	**66,470**

Source: Author's calculations using data from Project to Improve Financial Reporting and Auditing and annual budget statement.

---

[44] This includes allocations for both current and development streams.

Other pooled funds include the SHPI, which is funded by government revenues. Federal and provincial governments, military, cantonment boards, and autonomous bodies provide variable levels of health services coverage to their employees and dependents using government revenues. In addition, **private voluntary health insurance covers only 0.3% of the province's population**, while the Employees Social Security Institution, through a compulsory health insurance scheme for private entities with more than 10 employees, provides coverage to 1.3% of the population. There are a few smaller pools providing coverage to the informal sector, especially the poor and vulnerable (see Appendix 7 for an overview of the segments of the population from the formal and informal sectors receiving partial or comprehensive health services).

If all stated coverages are realized (for instance, the 69% coverage of the population through SHPI) and assuming no overlap between population segments, then about 95% of the population will be entitled to some form of health coverage by the end of 2018 (Figure 9). **However, the fragmented pooling architecture may result in overlapping coverage for some services, while other needed health services might be overlooked, especially for the vulnerable.** Moreover, for the health care providers, it may be confusing and inefficient working with various, possibly contending, purchasing agencies. Nonetheless, there are several initiatives on which UHC can be further built.

Figure 9: National Health Accounts, 2015–2016

% of total population covered

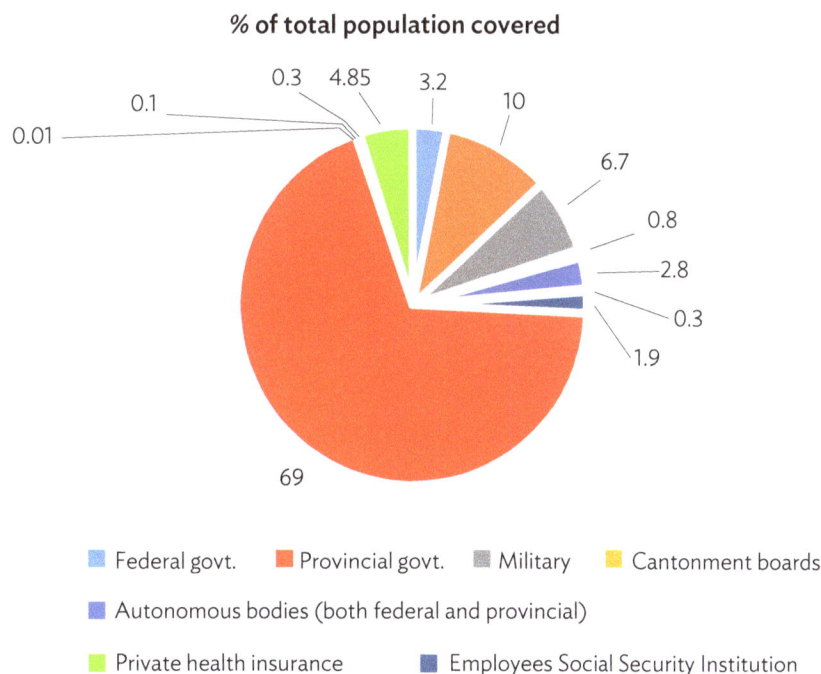

Legend:
- Federal govt.
- Provincial govt.
- Military
- Cantonment boards
- Autonomous bodies (both federal and provincial)
- Private health insurance
- Employees Social Security Institution

Source: Government of Khyber Pakhtunkhwa, Department of Finance. 2017.

Purchasing

Purchasing of health services in Khyber Pakhtunkhwa is fragmented. Federal and provincial health systems, military, Employees Social Security Institution, autonomous bodies, and cantonment boards directly provide services through their own facilities. The federal government has been financing national vertical programs at the provincial level, and a few dedicated programs for illnesses, like cancer and diabetes, have been recently initiated by the provincial government. The private sector has created an incentive for employment by combining profit-sharing mechanisms with salaries; fee for service is the predominant payment mechanism.

With regard to **how the provincial government purchases with its budget or allocates its budget to line items**, 55% of the 2018 budget (PRs36.07 billion or $311.93 million) was for employee-related expenses. There are decreased allocations for civil works at $24.65 million in 2018 from $40.47 million in 2017, while the budget for repairs and maintenance remains low at $0.52 million (Table 12).

Table 12: Consolidated Allocations by Major Line Items

Budget Type	FY2017			FY2018		
	PRs billion	$ million	%	PRs billion	$ million	%
Employee-related expenses	27.65	239.12	50	36.07	311.93	55
Operating expenses	19.51	168.72	36	20.15	174.26	31
Grants[a]	1.52	13.14	3	1.85	16.00	3
Transfers[b]	1.45	12.54	3	3.04	26.29	5
Physical assets	0.07	0.60	0	2.00	17.30	3
Civil works	4.68	40.47	9	2.85	24.65	4
Repairs and maintenance	0.06	0.52	0	0.06	0.52	0
Total	**54.94**	**475.11**	**100**	**66.02**	**570.95**	**100**

Note: Percentages may not total 100% because of rounding.

[a] Grants are used for transferring money from the province to districts, making payments to the family of the deceased, paying subsidies, and writing off loans.
[b] Transfers are used to record scholarships (stipends to postgraduate trainees and others are also recorded here); pay international agencies, e.g., procurement of vaccines from UNICEF; and disburse entertainment and gifts.

Source: Government of Khyber Pakhtunkhwa, Department of Health. 2017. *Budget Brief 2017-18*.

Regarding the activities funded, **the largest component of the 2015–2016 health expenditures as reported in the National Health Accounts is the delivery of hospital services at 97%.** This signals the need to reallocate resources to primary care and public health services in Khyber Pakhtunkhwa (Table 13).

Table 13: Current Health Expenditures by Activities, 2015–2016

Activities	Federal	Punjab	Sindh	KP	Balochistan	Pakistan
			PRs million			
General services		2,208		20	685	2,913
Health administration	1,520	15,898	7,078	418	1,485	26,399
Hospital services	10,308	123,684	38,457	14,970	11,242	198,661
Medical products, appliances, and equipment	27		75	5	27	134
Public health services	417	4,406	3,090	23	368	8,304
R&D health						–
Construction and transport						–
Economic, commercial, and labor affairs						–
Transfers			446			446
Administration			11			11
Others			355	20	97	472
Total	**12,272**	**146,196**	**49,512**	**15,456**	**13,904**	**237,340**

KP = Khyber Pakhtunkhwa, R&D = research and development.

Source: Government of Pakistan, Pakistan Bureau of Statistics. 2018. *National Health Accounts Pakistan 2015-16.* Islamabad.

The budget for secondary health care facilities has increased more than 3.4 times over the last 5 years (from 2012–2013 to 2016–2017) (Table 14). However, the year-on-year increase in the budget has been erratic, as low as 7% (FY2015) and as high as 74% (FY2014). This inconsistent increase points to a weaker link between policy and budgeting. On average, 84% of the allocations were made for the district headquarters hospitals and 16% for the *tehsil* headquarters hospitals during the period analyzed.

Table 14: Consolidated Current Budget and Expenditure of Secondary Care Facilities (PRs in million)

Expenditure Type	2012–2013		2013–2014		2014–2015		2015–2016		2016–2017	
	B	E	B	E	B	E	B	E	B	E
Salaries	1,733.77	1,590.75	3,529.07	2,913.70	3,698.12	3,305.19	4,896.53	4,158.19	6,610.27	6,264.02
Operating expenses	347.57	331.71	842.46	698.14	1,131.15	1,018.70	1,334.27	1,137.39	1,255.14	1,071.58
Grants	16.17	16.16	9.20	6.80	9.21	7.90	8.00	5.40	13.30	8.57
Transfer payments	10.13	9.02	2.16	2.12	2.24	2.24	3.31	3.02	844.46	844.44
Physical assets	553.79	507.63	254.55	89.06	126.88	109.61	128.16	102.60	160.26	144.79
Repairs and maintenance	14.91	14.37	25.34	23.12	38.49	34.11	40.37	37.61	48.89	46.60
Total	**2,676.34**	**2,469.64**	**4,662.78**	**3,732.94**	**5,006.08**	**4,477.76**	**6,410.63**	**5,444.21**	**8,932.32**	**8,380.00**

B = budget, E = expenditure.

Note: Numbers may not sum precisely because of rounding.

Source: Author's calculation using data from Project to Improve Financial Reporting and Auditing.

Figure 10: Average Allocation (5 Years) by Items of Expenditure for Secondary Care Hospitals

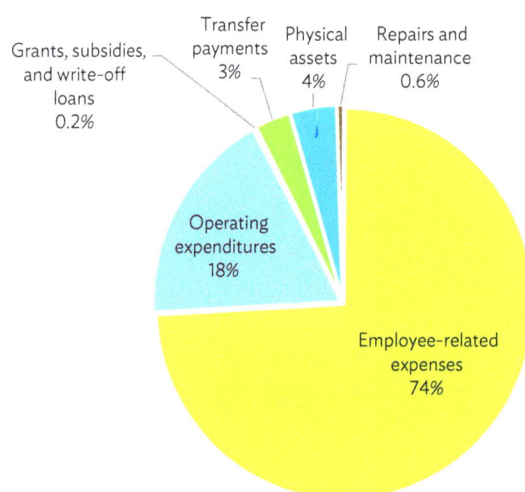

Grants, subsidies, and write-off loans 0.2%
Transfer payments 3%
Physical assets 4%
Repairs and maintenance 0.6%
Operating expenditures 18%
Employee-related expenses 74%

Note: Percentages may not total 100% because of rounding.

Source: Project to Improve Financial Reporting and Auditing.

The lion's share of the budget is the payment of salaries for the secondary health care facility staff at more than 74%. Repairs and maintenance during the last 5 years has received only 0.6% of the allocations (Figure 10).

There is an imbalance in the mix of expenditures that is purchased through the provincial health budget. The non-salary part impacts on the quality of service delivery, ensuring the delivery of services and continuation of operations. The major reason for the increase in overall allocations for the secondary health care facilities is the significant increase in salaries over the analyzed period, resulting in a growing imbalance between salary and non-salary allocations. The non-salary component has decreased its share from 35% in FY2013 to 23% in FY2017. Decreasing share of this level of expenditure category generates an inadequate supply of medicines, bedding, X-ray films, and other medical supplies, impacting on the quality, credibility, and reliability of services designed to be provided (Figure 11).

Figure 11: Expenditure Mix—Salary and Non-Salary (Secondary Health Care Facilities)

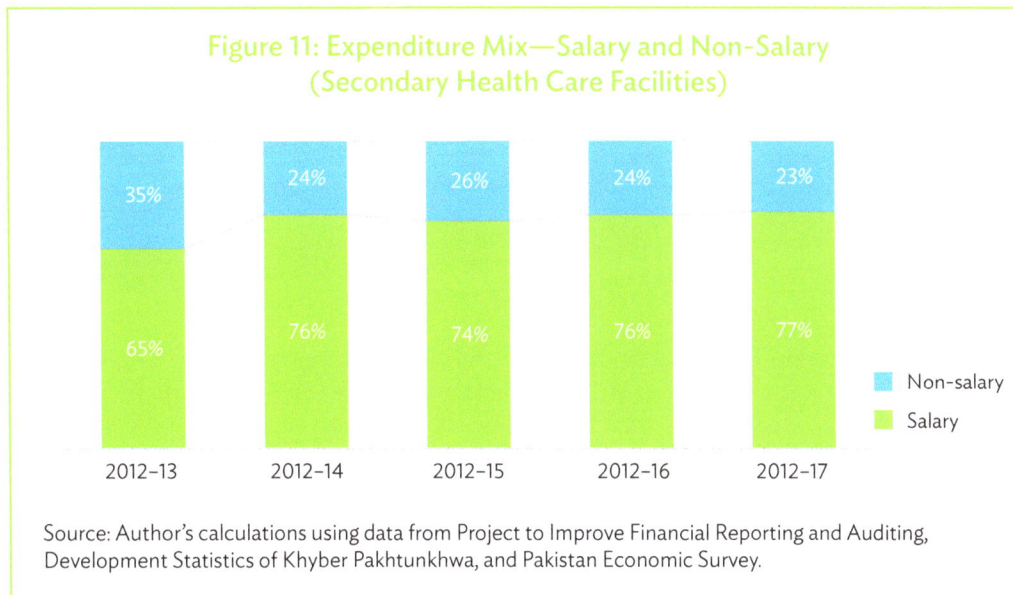

Year	Non-salary	Salary
2012–13	35%	65%
2012–14	24%	76%
2012–15	26%	74%
2012–16	24%	76%
2012–17	23%	77%

Source: Author's calculations using data from Project to Improve Financial Reporting and Auditing, Development Statistics of Khyber Pakhtunkhwa, and Pakistan Economic Survey.

However, a single-payer system also warrants a strong oversight mechanism. Such an oversight could be jointly performed by the Health Care Commission (HCC), which is responsible for the registration and quality assurance of private and public health care establishments, and the DOH.

On behalf of the Sehat Insaf Card holders, the SHPI purchases health services from more than 100 empaneled public and private hospitals, including MTIs and DHQ hospitals throughout the province, which represent around 53% of all hospitals (126 public and 63 private hospitals) providing inpatient services (footnote 35). To facilitate access to health care services, SLIC has established facilitation desks at prominent places in each empaneled hospital. The desks are branded and equipped with necessary information technology equipment and human resources.

For the empanelment of the hospitals, the SHPI-contracted SLIC assessed the available public and private health care facilities on a predefined criterion provided by the DOH. Empaneled government hospitals can retain, without diminution of their budget, a minimum of 75% of the insurance income from SHPI. The retained insurance funds can be utilized for the improvement of quality of health care services and payment of incentives to the hospital staff. About 25% of the fund to be remitted to the government can be accrued in the special account or health fund, established and used solely for enhancements in the insurance program. In parallel, there are ongoing MTI reforms, including comprehensive financial and management autonomy reforms, which can be models for further reforms in other empaneled government hospitals.

First, as the empanelment takes place, it becomes more apparent that health facilities cannot yet sufficiently deliver quality health services (footnote 17) due to a shortage of health facilities and medical and paramedical staff. Second, there is a disconnect between supply and demand for health care (for instance, there is inflexibility in shifting beds from one department to another, where there is high demand). And third, improvements are required in quality of care.

Furthermore, as the population coverage of SHPI expands to 69% of the poorest population of Khyber Pakhtunkhwa, there is a need to determine the appropriate premium amount to ensure that only inpatient care requiring hospitalization is purchased and also outpatient care including medicines and diagnostics prescribed during the visits. A preliminary actuarial study provides preliminary cost estimates and supply and demand, but this needs to be deepened (Appendix 9).

IV.   Recommendations

Increase Revenue Collection and Strengthen Government Purchasing

- Moving toward UHC in Khyber Pakhtunkhwa requires increased revenue collection that would increase the share of prepayments for health while reducing the share of household OOP health expenditure. It needs to reduce the fragmentation of the different prepayment pools, particularly the provincial health budget and the SHPI. It needs to strengthen government purchasing including coordination in the budgetary allocation of the provincial health budget and the health services purchased by SHPI.
- Increased space for tax collection in Pakistan and Khyber Pakhtunkhwa allows more budget for health sector. Funds can be generated through increasing the general taxation or improved collection. They can either be made available through federal transfers, or through direct financing support through the cost-sharing of the premium subsidies for SHPI members and sharing in the financing of health sector civil works construction or upgrading.
- The Federal Ministry of NHSRC, **while planning the implementation and earmarking mechanisms for the sin tax on cigarettes and sugary beverages**, can learn from sin tax reforms in Ghana, Iran, and the Philippines, where part of the value-added tax collections is used to pay for the subsidized health insurance premiums of the eligible population.
- **The consolidation of the Employees Social Security Institution, Zakat, Bait-ul-Mal, and other schemes into the SHPI** will not only increase revenues but also reduce fragmentation and strengthen the purchasing power of SHPI. After this initial set of consolidation, bringing together the budget line items of the provincial health department and district governments used for hospital service delivery with the SHPI can be considered. Once all these prepaid funds are pooled under SHPI, fragmentation

will be reduced to a minimum, and government purchasing becomes stronger. However, SHPI purchasing can only do so much if the current health infrastructure of Khyber Pakhtunkhwa remains inadequate to deliver the health services needed by the population. The actuarial analysis shows that the Government of Khyber Pakhtunkhwa and the private sector need to invest in the health care infrastructure to assure continuous supply-side readiness, especially once enrolled members start consuming their benefits under SHPI. Building up the capacity of both government and private health care providers to work with health insurers is also needed.

Improve Public Financial Management

As supply-side readiness improves, SHPI needs to focus on primary care and not just hospital care services. As it becomes the main government purchaser in Khyber Pakhtunkhwa, SHPI must purchase the health services and goods that are most needed. This action requires ensuring that the government and SHPI have the skills and capabilities to do costing of health services, conduct health technology assessments, manage contracts (both with SLIC and the empaneled hospitals), and deploy and use digital health interventions. It also requires improved public financial management (PFM) practices by government hospitals, such as the following:

- **Improving the planning and budgeting capacity both at district and provincial levels by increasing the number of skilled workers.** This includes identifying the capacity gaps at both levels. This should also keep in mind the expanding role in financial management that can be given to the secondary care health facilities especially for insurance reimbursements.
- **Supporting the process of budget development** and linking it with policy using the Health Sector Strategy (HSS) as a guiding document, done both at district and provincial levels.
- **Automating budgeting and expenditure reporting systems** to improve the efficiency of budgeting and expenditure monitoring.
- **Establishing regular routines to monitor budget execution** both for current and development budget streams, done at district and provincial levels.

References

Abdullah, Tanweer and Shaw. 2006. A Review of the Experience of Hospital Autonomy in Pakistan. *The International Journal of Health Planning and Management.* 22 (1). pp. 45–62.

ADB. 2017. *Key Indicators for Asia and the Pacific 2017.* Manila.

Ahmed, Nadeem and Yunis. 2011. *Institutionalizing Quality in Health Care of Khyber Pakhtunkhwa: A Process of Sustaining Change.* Presentation at the 12th International Convention on Quality Improvement. Lahore, Pakistan. 2–3 May.

S. Amjad. 2014: *Final Evaluation: Chitral Child Survival Project, Chitral, Khyber Pakhtunkhwa, Pakistan.* Islamabad: United States Agency for International Development / Aga Khan Foundation. https://pdf.usaid.gov/pdf_docs/pa00k2gc.pdf.

C. Cashin et al. 2017. Aligning Public Financial Management and Health Financing: Sustaining Progress Toward Universal Health Coverage. *Health Financing Working Paper.* No. 4. Geneva: World Health Organization.

S. Cevik. 2016. Unlocking Pakistan's Revenue Potential. *IMF Working Paper.* No. 16/182. Washington, DC: International Monetary Fund.

A. Faisel. 2012. *Minimum Health Services Delivery Package for Primary Health Care Facilities in Khyber Pakhtunkhwa.* Lahore: Technical Resource Facility.

Financial Cooperation between the Federal Republic of Germany and the Islamic Republic of Pakistan; BMZ no 2013 66 228: Preparatory Study for the Social Health Protection Project Phase II; Final Report, management4health, Frankfurt am Main, September 2017.

F. Finkelstein et al. 2009. PD in the Developing World: Peritoneal Dialysis in the Developing World: Recommendations from a Symposium at the ISPD Meeting 2008. *International Society for Peritoneal Dialysis.* 29 (6). pp. 618–622.

Government of Khyber Pakhtunkhwa, DOH. 2010. *Health Sector Strategy 2010–2017.* Pakistan.

Government of Khyber Pakhtunkhwa, DOH. 2016. Notification No. PO-IV/H/6-7/SHPI/2016 on the allocation of the Health Insurance Fund.

Government of Khyber Pakhtunkhwa, DOH. 2017. *Budget Brief 2017-18*. http://www.healthkp.gov.pk/wp-content/uploads/2017/11/Health-Budget-Brief-FY2017-18-DOH.pdf.

Government of Khyber Pakhtunkhwa, DOH. 2017. *Khyber Pakhtunkhwa Health Survey 2017*. http://www.healthkp.gov.pk/wpcontent/uploads/2017/12/KPHS2017_30_Oct_2017.pdf.

Government of Khyber Pakhtunkhwa, Planning and Development Department, Bureau of Statistics. 2017. *Development Statistics of Khyber Pakhtunkhwa 2017*. Pakistan.

Government of Pakistan, Ministry of National Health Services, Regulations and Coordination. 2012. *National Nutrition Survey 2011*. Islamabad.

Government of Pakistan, Pakistan Bureau of Statistics. 2018. *National Health Accounts Pakistan 2015-16*. Islamabad.

H. Huitzing. 2018. *Actuarial Model for the Supply and Demand Side Interventions in the Khyber Pakhtunkhwa Health Sector*. Background paper for the Assessment of the Khyber Pakhtunkhwa Health Sector. Peshawar. 13–15 February.

W. Hulrbut and M. Caroline, eds. 2002. *The Next Ascent: An Evaluation of the Aga Khan Rural Support Program*. Washington, DC: World Bank.

Institute of Medicine. 2000. *To Err is Human: Building a Safer Health System*. Washington, DC: The National Academies Press.

Jain, Arsh, Blake, Cordy and Garg. 2012. Global Trends in Rates of Peritoneal Dialysis. *Journal of the American Society of Nephrology*. 23 (3). pp. 533–544.

B. Loevinsohn. 2006. Partnering with NGOs to Strengthen Management: An External Evaluation of the Chief Minister's Initiative on Primary Health Care in Rahim Yar Khan District, Punjab. *South Asia Human Development Sector Series*. No. 13. Washington, DC: World Bank.

A. Mahmood. 2018. *Public Financial Management Assessment: Health Sector*. Background paper for the Assessment of the Khyber Pakhtunkhwa Health Sector. Peshawar. 13–15 February.

J. Martinez et al. 2010. *Third-Party Evaluation of the PPHI in Pakistan: Findings, Conclusions and Recommendations*. Lahore: Technical Resource Facility / Health and Life Sciences Partnership.

Ministry of Health, Directorate General Health Services, Khyber Pakhtunkhwa, Peshawar: District Health Information System (DHIS)—Annual Report 2017 www.dhiskp.gov.pk/reports/Annual%20Report%202017%20N.pdf.

I. Nasir. 2018. *Drug Regulation*. Background paper for the Assessment of the Khyber Pakhtunkhwa Health Sector. Peshawar. 13–15 February.

National Institute of Population Studies and ICF International. 2013. *Pakistan Demographic and Health Survey 2012-13*. Islamabad.

F. Ng. 2018. *Khyber Pakhtunkhwa Planning for Physical and Human Resources*. Background paper for the Assessment of the Khyber Pakhtunkhwa Health Sector. Peshawar. 13–15 February.

M. Niechzial. 2018. *Challenges and Solutions for Better Quality*. Background paper for the Assessment of the Khyber Pakhtunkhwa Health Sector. Peshawar. 13–15 February.

S. Nishtar. 2010. *Choked Pipes: Reforming Pakistan's Mixed Health System*. Oxford, United Kingdom: Oxford University Press.

A. Saeed. 2013. Understanding Policy Making and Implementation in Pakistan: A Case of Hospital Autonomy Reforms. *Public Policy and Administration Research*. 3 (1).

Secondary Care Standards for Quality Health Services in NWFP, GTZ (Deutsche Gesellschaft für Internationale Zusammenarbeit), January 2007.

Siddiq, Aqsa, Balioch and Takrim. *Confidential Evaluation Report for Clinical & Performance Audit of MTI-Hayatabad Medical Complex*. Islamabad.

Siddiq, Aqsa, Balioch and Takrim. 2016. Quality of Healthcare Services in Public and Private Hospitals of Peshawar, Pakistan: A Comparative Study Using SERVQUAL. *City University Research Journal*. 6 (2). pp. 242–255.

Thaver, Inayat and Khalid. 2016. *Final Report: Secondary Level Minimum Health Services Delivery Package for Secondary Care Hospitals (MHSDP)*.

The Kidney Foundation. 2014. *Dialysis Registry of Pakistan 2014*. http://www.kidneyfoundation.net.pk/KF_Book.pdf.

United Nations Development Programme. 2014. *Development Advocate Pakistan*. Volume 1, Issue 1, https://www.undp.org/content/dam/pakistan/docs/DevelopmentPolicy/dev%20final%20versions.pdf.

Wajid, Gohar, Al Zarouni and Al Massoud. 2002. *Healthcare Quality Improvement in Pakistani Hospitals*. Paper presented at the 7th International Convention on Quality Improvement. Karachi, Pakistan. 26–27 October.

World Health Organization. 2018. *Handbook for National Quality Policy and Strategy: A Practical Approach for Developing Policy and Strategy to Improve Quality of Care*. Geneva.

World Health Organization. 2006. Chapter 1: Health Workers: A Global Profile. In *Working Together for Health: The World Health Report 2006*. Geneva.

World Health Organization. 2010. *Monitoring the Building Blocks of Health Systems: A Handbook of Indicators and Their Measurement Strategies*. Geneva.

World Health Organization. 2010. Chapter 4: More Health for the Money. In *The World Health Report: Health Systems Financing: The Path to Universal Coverage*. Geneva.

World Health Organization. Health Financing for Universal Coverage. http://www.who.int/health_financing/topics/fiscal-space/main-drivers/en/.

Zaidi et al. 2015. Can Contracted Out Health Facilities Improve Access, Equity, and Quality of Maternal and Newborn Health Services? Evidence from Pakistan. *Health Research Policy and Systems*. 13 (Suppl 1): 54.

Appendixes

Appendix 1—Case Study on Hospital Contracting Experience in Khyber Pakhtunkhwa

Strategic Priorities: Contracting in Medical Teaching Institutions

Hospital autonomy has a long history in Pakistan, dating back to the mid-1990s in Punjab,[1] but it has faced many ups and downs over time. In Khyber Pakhtunkhwa, it started in 2000 when the four large teaching hospitals—Lady Reading Hospital, Khyber Teaching Hospital, Hayatabad Medical Complex Peshawar, and Ayub Teaching Hospital—were given autonomy. More recently, the Government of Khyber Pakhtunkhwa has reframed the autonomy of these hospitals under Medical Teaching Institutions (MTI) Act, 2015, considering whether to make secondary hospitals more autonomous. It has also contracted out the management and operation of certain primary health care (PHC) facilities. This case study looks at the province's experience in autonomy and contracting out health service provision often under a public–private partnership (PPP) arrangement, and then discusses the current status of secondary hospitals concerning governance and management and assessing the potential for autonomizing secondary hospitals.

As previously stated, MTIs (the large teaching hospitals) have been given formal managerial and financial autonomy. They enjoy extended autonomy including the ability to set their user fees. They now depend on the central provincial government rather than the Department of Health (DOH). Their experience, although still recent, is relevant to the discussion of autonomy for secondary hospitals because it represents the only experience of full formal autonomy in Khyber Pakhtunkhwa health facilities, and several lessons are to be learned from that experience.

While their autonomous status has given them full latitude to improve efficiency and quality in service delivery, it has also been criticized on several grounds. It is worth noting that the autonomy has been given to the MTI as a whole, of which the hospitals are a part. All MTIs have a board of governors, which is responsible for the strategic planning and management of both the college and the hospital. The Government of Khyber Pakhtunkhwa appoints their members based on recommendations of a special search and nomination council. However, the composition of these boards is questionable, as all the members are from the private sector and have limited

---

[1] A. Saeed. 2013. Understanding Policy Making and Implementation in Pakistan: A Case of Hospital Autonomy Reforms. Public Policy and Administration Research. 3 (1).

or no health background. The DOH representatives are members of the council but do not participate in the board. The board then appoints a dean of the MTI, a hospital director, and a medical director.

The teaching hospital is accountable to the board, who in turn is accountable to the Government of Khyber Pakhtunkhwa for their performance based on monitoring and evaluation (M&E) and audits. However, the M&E framework has yet to be defined, and no instrument (e.g., a contract) is in place to determine service and performance goals, indicators, and standards.

Practically, the governance and management structure of MTI hospitals is split between four directors—hospital director (management functions), medical director (medical functions), nursing director (nursing affairs), finance director (financial affairs)—and the college of the attached university (which employs all physicians). All are appointed by and report to the board, which does not necessarily have members with a health or hospital background. The interests and goals of the two entities and the various profession-based directors are often conflicting, and educational priorities often prevail over service delivery and management. Although MTIs are supposed to follow government's health policies, there is no clear channel of communication between the hospital and the DOH, and thus no way for the DOH to provide policy guidance or technical oversight. Private practice and fee charging are allowed in MTI premises, and the MTIs may set these fees and retain all fee revenue for internal use.

Shifa Foundation undertook performance audits on the MTIs in 2017. These performance audits were limited by two factors that prevented measuring progress since autonomization: (i) the time since the act had come into force was limited (2 years); (ii) the audits were based on the Joint Commission International standards for accreditation, and thus emphasized clinical aspects and quality of care. Evaluation was made against absolute international standards rather than improvements relative to the situation before the autonomy act or comparisons with other hospitals in Khyber Pakhtunkhwa. Given that the assessment was made against standards in several areas, it is difficult to draw general conclusions. Nonetheless, their findings are relevant and point to both strengths and weaknesses of the MTIs. Clinical processes were established but insufficiently standardized. No quality improvement program was in place, although there were several quality initiatives. Initiatives in management functions (including information systems) took place but were hardly part of an overall plan and strategy. Standard operating procedures (SOPs) were found in some areas but not in others. MTIs hired staff directly to fill gaps. Revenue from user fees increased substantially (33% from 2015 to 2016 in Hayatabad Medical Complex Peshawar). The audits did not assess efficiency in resource allocation and use or accountability.

Contracting Out for Primary Health Care and Hospital Services

Over the years the Government of Khyber Pakhtunkhwa has contracted out the management and/or the provision of primary and hospital services to various private organizations, usually nongovernment organizations (NGOs) or charity organizations. These contracts include the PPP arrangements with Aga Khan Foundation (and Aga Khan Health Services), the largest nonprofit organization in Pakistan, for the management of hospitals and primary health care (PHC) in the remote Chitral District. Aga Khan has similar arrangements in other provinces including Sindh, Baltistan, and Punjab. The contracts also include the People´s Primary Healthcare Initiative (PPHI) experience in PHC. While systematic evaluations of these experiences have not been done, a few focused audit and evaluation reports are available, and field visits can provide some insights.

The Aga Khan Foundation project in Chitral (2008–2014) was assessed in a 2014 report funded by the United States Agency for International Development. According to the report, comparing a set of indicators before and after the project indicated that "the project has achieved remarkable results in terms of overall outcomes and outputs particularly in improving skilled birth attendance, continuum of care and increasing use of maternal care services by women."[2] Managerial and quality processes had also improved substantially, but concerns were raised regarding the continuity of these improvements after the end of the project.[3] Another earlier report arrived at similar results.[4]

An assessment of the PPHI experience in Khyber Pakhtunkhwa and other provinces was performed in 2010 to evaluate the impact of this model in comparison with traditionally publicly provided PHC services. The findings are as follows: "It is quite clear that in the districts where PPHI has been operating for the longest time (approximately 2 years since mid or end 2007 until January 2010) PPHI has achieved significant improvements in staffing, availability of drugs and equipment and physical condition of facilities, including rehabilitation and repossession of hitherto dysfunctional BHUs. Improvements have also been measured by the third-party evaluation in terms of services delivered (outpatient, antenatal care attendance, and consumer satisfaction)".[5] The study identifies the autonomy for hiring additional staff, resource allocation, and stronger supervision as key factors in generating positive results. It also points out the weakness of the contracting arrangement used with respect to scope (service package to be provided), institutional relations and responsibilities between the contractor and contractee, oversight, and performance M&E (footnote 4). The report suggests that most of the limitations encountered arise from the unsupportive context in which the model has operated and the weakness of the contracting instrument and of the contractor's capacity for contract management and M&E. Other studies looking at other projects have reached similar conclusions.[6]

In spite of some limitations in the number, scope, and methodological design of some evaluations, available evidence suggests that these experiences of health PPPs or contracting out health service provision have been mostly successful. However, the DOH senior staff do not necessarily support these conclusions, and there is widespread resistance to these innovative models both within DOH and in society at large. Many such projects have been discontinued, apparently for political reasons or short-term considerations. For example, the PPHI contract has been discontinued in late 2017. A major issue that is often pointed to, though, is the limited capacity of the DOH for preparing, negotiating, monitoring, and evaluating these contracts, as well as the lack of continued political support for the projects.

Evidence from the Field (Primary Health Care Facilities and Secondary Hospitals)

Health facilities, especially hospitals, enjoy variable levels of autonomy depending on the type of facility and the managerial area of interest. They are broadly responsible for their procurement

---

[2]   S. Amjad. 2014: *Final Evaluation: Chitral Child Survival Project, Chitral, Khyber Pakhtunkhwa, Pakistan.* Islamabad: United States Agency for International Development / Aga Khan Foundation. https://pdf.usaid.gov/pdf_docs/pa00k2gc.pdf.

[3]   The report focused on the maternal and child health component; no assessment of the Chitral Hospital project could be found.

[4]   W. Hurlbut and C. McEuen, eds. 2002: *The Next Ascent: An Evaluation of the Aga Khan Rural Support Program.* Washington, DC: World Bank.

[5]   J. Martinez et al. 2010. *Third-Party Evaluation of the PPHI in Pakistan: Findings, Conclusions and Recommendations.* Lahore: Technical Resource Facility / Health and Life Sciences Partnership.

[6]   S. Zaidi et al. 2015. Can Contracted Out Health Facilities Improve Access, Equity, and Quality of Maternal and Newborn Health Services? Evidence from Pakistan. *Health Research Policy and Systems.* 13 (Suppl 1): 54.

and budget preparation, but district-level facilities have no authority for reallocating the line item budget or for hiring and firing staff. The budgeting process is formally bottom-up, but facility managers have no information on the budget envelope in the preparation phase, and the final approved budget is often quite different from the proposal made by the facilities.

A striking feature in field visits to various health facilities is the wide variation in facility infrastructure, operations, management, and process quality. While MTI hospitals usually are well staffed and have reasonably organized processes and management, smaller hospitals management is often found to be very weak or ineffective. This weakness seems to be closely correlated with its management status and model, as well as the level of the facility. In autonomized MTIs (large teaching hospitals), infrastructure, management, and clinical processes are much better than in lower-level hospitals. Facilities managed by private partners through some PPPs are better supervised and in better shape than facilities under direct public management (under the DOH or district health authorities), although formal evaluations are scarce. Within the public sector, lower-level facilities are usually worse off; this could be related to a de facto prioritization of higher-level hospitals in resource allocation; the inability to secure and retain trained facility managers in small, remote facilities; or both.

To strengthen both autonomy and accountability of public facilities, the Government of Khyber Pakhtunkhwa has promoted the establishment of facility boards in many facilities. Of the facilities covered in our survey, 16 (43%) had a board in place, and 21 did not. However, the functionality and effectiveness of these boards vary substantially. Four boards met less than quarterly during the last year, while seven met more than monthly, and one was created but not operational (Table A1).

The actual role of these facility boards is unclear and seems to vary across facilities. Generally, the facility boards are supposed to provide both some autonomy in raising and managing alternative sources of funds and an accountability body close to the facility operations. However, the membership of the boards is not adequate for effective strategic, supervision, and accountability functions. Most members are private sector businessmen, and thus expected to provide independent guidance and accountability to facility managers, but are often not familiar with the goals, policies, and constraints of the health sector and public management. They are also not immune to political pressures. Moreover, no community representatives are present in the boards, which prevent the community served by the facility to have a say in strategic management or evaluation of the facilities.

Secondary hospitals enjoy limited real managerial and financial autonomy. They prepare and submit their annual budget and plan, but the final decision on budget level and allocation is made by the DOH and is often quite different from the proposed budget.

Hospitals raise their revenue from user fees and insurance reimbursements. The DOH issued a recent notification defining that insurance payments should be retained at the facility at the level of 75% (the remaining 25% are to be deposited at the health insurance fund account at the provincial level). The notification also defines specific percentages for spending these revenues (60% for quality improvement, 25% for medical staff, 10% for nursing staff, 3% for repair expenses, and 2% for administrative staff).

Table A1: Status of Facility Boards

Facility Type	No. of Meetings						Not Functional	No Board
	2	3	4	5–6	7–12	>12		
Teaching hospitals						2		
Specialized hospitals					1		1	2
DHQ hospitals	1	1	1			1		4
THQ hospitals					1	2		9
Other hospitals						1		2
RHCs				1	1			2
Dispensaries								1
Mother and child health centers								1
Other outpatient facilities			1			1		
Total	1	1	2	1	3	7	1	21

DHQ = district headquarters, RHC = rural health center, THQ = *tehsil* headquarters.

Source: Government of Khyber Pakhtunkhwa, Department of Health. 2017.

Conclusion: Hospital Autonomy from a Governance Perspective

The discussion of previous and current experiences of hospital autonomy in Khyber Pakhtunkhwa reveals structural weaknesses that relate to the World Health Organization (WHO) framework. First, there is not at present a clear institutional design for health facility autonomy, and autonomy initiatives have been mostly launched ad hoc. Second, there is no clear general policy on autonomy or implementation plan. Third, the regulatory framework relating to facility autonomy is weak and inconsistent, which allows potentially rich initiatives to be challenged legally and disrupted or discontinued. Fourth, as discussed above, hospital autonomy has not been supported by a clear and strong accountability system, which prompts the Ministry of National Health Services, Regulations and Coordination (NHSRC) to argue that it has "lost control" over autonomized hospitals and that it does not follow national policies and goals.

Appendix 2—Key Elements of a Strong Contract

The key elements of a strong contract are illustrated in Figure A1. The main distinction between a contract and a memorandum of understanding is that the contract has legal value and is therefore enforceable. The objectives of the contract and the roles and responsibilities of each party need to be explicitly stated. Penalties should be clearly defined for any contract breach, noncompliance, or nonperformance. The contract should also specify clear goals and targets within a certain time frame and ways to measure them. Finally, the amount and basis for payment should be clearly defined, i.e., the provider payment mechanism. Therefore, a strong contract should also specify how performance will be measured and how it will impact payment.

Performance-based payments to providers tend to have a positive impact on performance in general, and quality and efficiency in particular. The right part of Figure A1 shows an example of contract payment partially linked to performance: around third of the total payment comes from a fixed base per capita payment; a third is based on relevant adjustments (such as poverty levels and health status across regions); and the last third is based on a predefined set of key performance indicators such as bed occupation and rotation, productivity of health personnel, and accreditation status or other quality-related indicators.

While contract management is a must in public–private partnerships (PPPs), contracted services, and autonomous hospitals, the Department of Health (DOH) could gradually move toward establishing some form of contract with public facilities in general to offer clear incentives for public providers to improve performance.

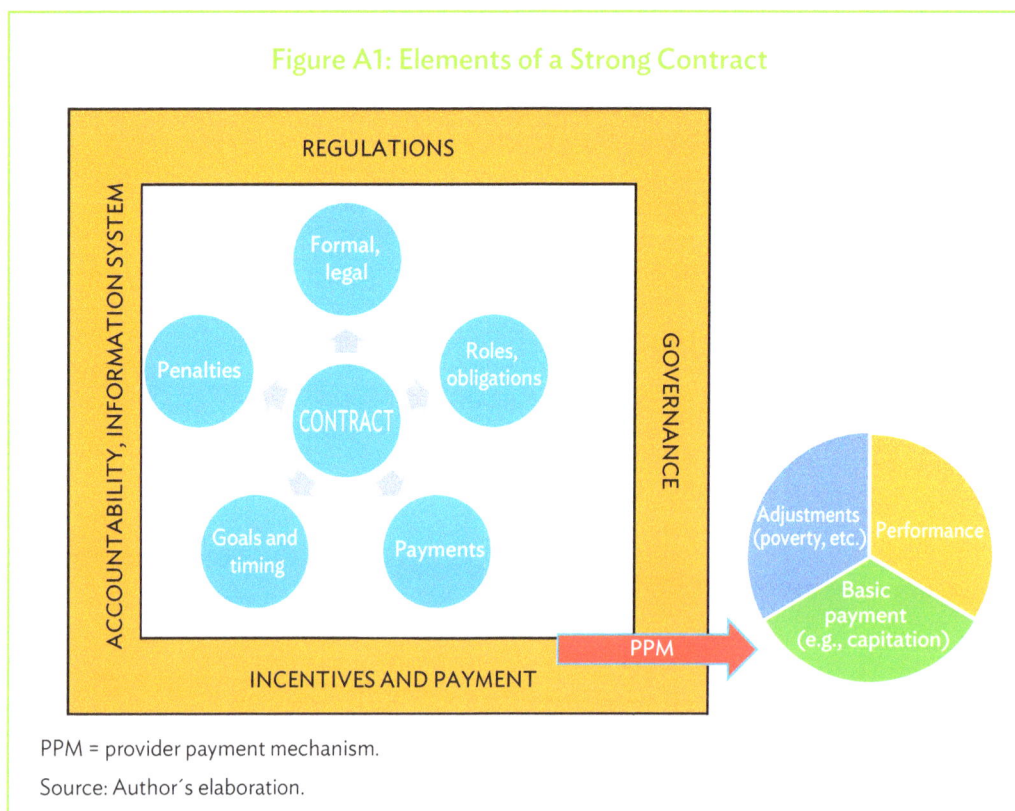

Figure A1: Elements of a Strong Contract

PPM = provider payment mechanism.

Source: Author´s elaboration.

Appendix 3—Methodology for Modeling Demand for Health Care

Using a population growth-based adjusted model to predict the health service and human resources for health (HRH) needs, the potential and relative gaps in resources to deliver health services through 2035 are enumerated across Khyber Pakhtunkhwa's districts. The methodology can be summarized in the following diagram:

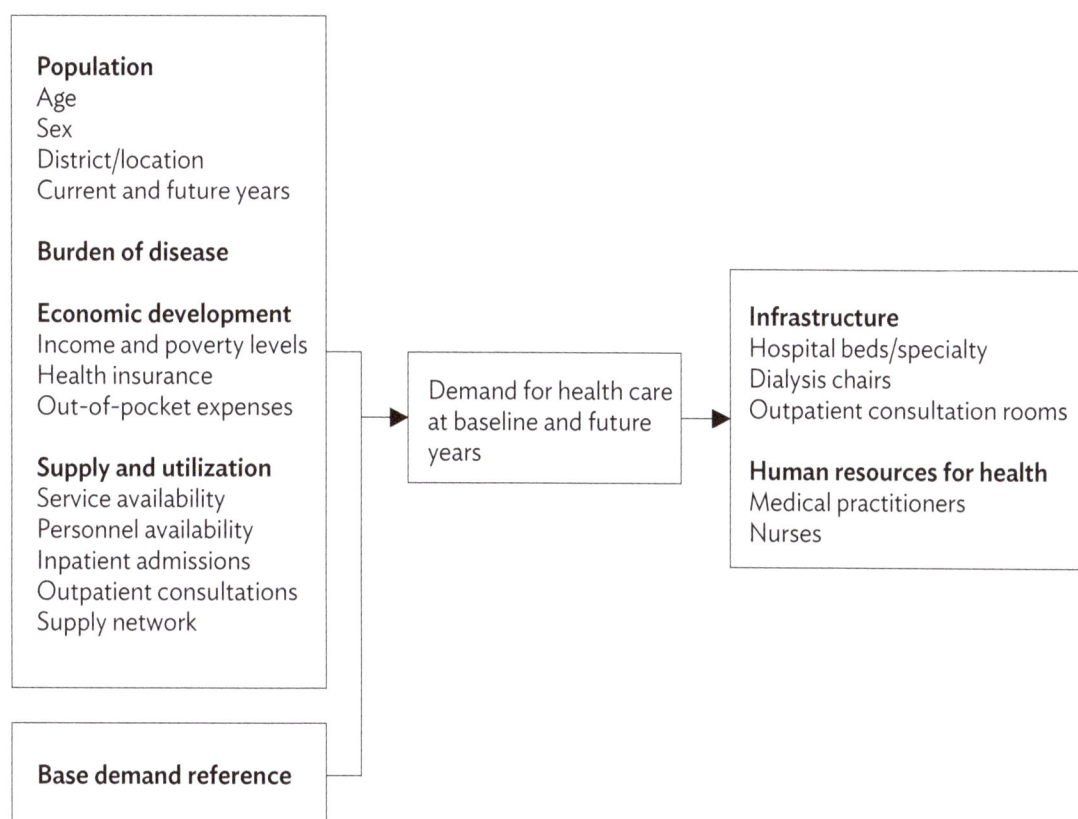

Population
Age
Sex
District/location
Current and future years

Burden of disease

Economic development
Income and poverty levels
Health insurance
Out-of-pocket expenses

Supply and utilization
Service availability
Personnel availability
Inpatient admissions
Outpatient consultations
Supply network

Base demand reference

Demand for health care at baseline and future years

Infrastructure
Hospital beds/specialty
Dialysis chairs
Outpatient consultation rooms

Human resources for health
Medical practitioners
Nurses

Source: Author's elaboration.

Appendix 4—Continuous Quality Improvement Description and Good Practice Examples of Standard Operating Procedures for Medical Care

Continuous Quality Improvement

The following elements are critical to implementing a sustainable quality management system leading to continuous quality improvement (CQI):

- Continuous capacity building will strengthen knowledge and skills development in the implementation (standards development, process improvement, etc.) and administration (leadership, planning, monitoring, etc.) of quality management activities.
- Regular information and communication on quality issues requiring investment in information and monitoring and evaluation (M&E) systems that measure and report on quality indicators will allow for regular analysis of the current situation and trends both at operational and governance levels.
- Recognizing and rewarding individual and team efforts will motivate health staff and managers to persevere in their efforts to meet client needs most effectively and efficiently.
- Facilitating the implementation of operational quality standards (guidelines and pathways) will help create the basis for a better organization and functioning of clinical services and lead to predictable results at the point of service delivery. Capacities for the implementation of standards need to be developed at all levels of the health care or hospital sector. Specific budgets should be made available to health facilities for quality improvement measures.
- Ways should be explored to involve the patient's perspective in a systemic quality management approach (e.g., through the introduction of a patient relations officer, ombudsman, or mediator position in all hospitals).

The standards documents (i) *Secondary Health Care Standards for Quality Health Services Volumes I–IV* developed in the framework of a Deutsche Gesellschaft für Internationale Zusammenarbeit technical assistance project and published in 2007, and (ii) *Secondary Level Minimum Health Services Delivery Package for Secondary Care Hospitals (MHSDP)* published in 2016 focus on structural elements of care (buildings, equipment, drugs, consumables, and human resources) as well as related management processes required to provide care to the patient and operate hospitals (clinical and support services). However, they do not contain any clinical (disease, syndrome, or symptom specific) guideline, protocol, or pathway (algorithm), describing the diagnostic and therapeutic measures to be undertaken in a patient who presents, or who is being admitted with, any of these symptoms, syndromes, or specific diseases or health problems.

Having these structural standards for buildings and equipment and general processes for service organization and management is already an important step. What needs to be done is to harmonize and operationalize these standards (nobody at facility level was even aware of their existence), i.e., to systematically analyze and evaluate compliance with these standards of all hospitals. This could and should be a precondition for licensing or accreditation of both public and private hospitals.

What is further needed is the elaboration of clinical guidelines and care protocols for the most frequent diseases and medical conditions that would require admission to secondary level inpatient care (targeting coverage of around 85% of the volume of services provided at this level). Usually the 10 most frequent diseases or conditions of all four basic disciplines—internal medicine, pediatrics, surgery, and gynecology or obstetrics—are sufficient to reach this target.

The following steps shall be undertaken:

1. Establish expert committees for each of the abovementioned core disciplines, e.g., teachers at the medical faculty of the University of Peshawar plus heads of departments and senior specialists of secondary level hospitals in Khyber Pakhtunkhwa. The number of members in each group shall be limited to 12 (four university experts plus eight heads of departments and senior specialist doctors of secondary health care hospitals). Each committee shall elect a chair, vice-chair (both representing the two different levels of care), and secretary. The committees may engage external experts or support for the development of specific protocols.
2. Define the list of diseases or conditions requiring inpatient care at secondary level hospitals based on existing facility, health management information system (HMIS) reports and statistics, and expert opinion.
3. Elaborate protocols for the 10 most frequent diseases or medical conditions requiring secondary level inpatient care (this process may take up to 1 year).
4. Introduce these protocols at pilot hospitals incrementally as they become available and are adopted by the DOH, preferably those hospitals that are represented in the committee through individual department heads and senior specialist doctors. Experience with the implementation shall be summarized in an evaluation report (to be developed for each pilot hospital) and lead to systematic review and adaptation and improvement of the first draft of the protocols. This process may take another 1 year, so that after 2 years final versions of these protocols shall be ready for rollout to all public and private hospitals. Compliance with these protocols as minimum quality standards shall become mandatory for all health care providers. However, providers may translate the general protocols into clinical pathways considering specificities in terms of infrastructure, equipment, human resources, etc. prevailing at their respective facilities.
5. Undertake a systematic review of all protocols every second year to make sure they still represent state-of-the-art knowledge and recommendations for diagnostic and therapeutic measures. The DOH (quality department) shall manage the process with technical support from the guideline committees. Members of the committees may be exchanged while maintaining the representativeness of the two levels of service delivery. It shall be noted that the protocols and pathways to be developed shall include guidelines for patient referral at both interfaces of secondary care: back to primary health care (PHC) level and forward to tertiary-level facilities.

Framework for Continuous Quality Improvement

Currently, no framework exists to promote quality of care at secondary hospitals in Khyber Pakhtunkhwa. The abovementioned protocols would be one element only. Two pillars need to be built to create a comprehensive framework for CQI—which is the ultimate objective of quality management in any sector—not only at service or facility level but also at the provincial level of the health care system: (i) internal quality management (clinical protocols and pathways), (ii) and external quality management (benchmarking with hospitals of the same level). Box A1 shows the World Health Organization Health Systems Framework and Quality of Care.

Both systems are based on continuous monitoring and evaluation of quality indicators demonstrating the following:

(i)   service performance—number of patients treated by diagnosis, different kinds of surgery undertaken, bed occupancy rate, average length of stay (ALOS) by diagnosis or kind of treatment;

(ii)   risk management or patient safety aspects—rates of hospital-acquired infections in general and postsurgical wound infection rate in particular, thrombosis or thromboembolism that occur during inpatient treatment, patient falls (with injury), readmission for the same diagnosis and/or related complications within less than 15 days, any case of inpatient mortality that shall be classified into avoidable and unavoidable cases; and

(iii) outcomes of medical treatment (usually in the framework of medium- to long-term follow-up evaluations)—survival of patients admitted with acute myocardial infarction or cerebrovascular insult (separate analysis of deaths occurring within first 24 hours from those occurring later), readmission of patients with diabetes or chronic obstructive pulmonary disease or asthma within less than 30 days after discharge, patient satisfaction (based on standard questionnaire) at discharge.

The above indicators are only examples based on international best practices. Other more appropriate indicators for the Pakistan and particularly Khyber Pakhtunkhwa context of secondary level care may be developed and added or replace less adequate ones. It is evident that timely and reliable collection of data and analysis of these indicators will depend on the availability of a functional hospital information system including electronic patient record (EPR). EPR may also help in introducing and sustaining the abovementioned standard operating procedures (SOPs) (predefined algorithms for diagnostic and therapeutic procedures laid down in the EPR system) and improving quality of care or avoiding risks, specifically those related to the application of drugs and other medical products (notification of allergies and incompatibilities between products, need to adapt dosage in patients with reduced renal or hepatic clearance, age-related adaptation of drug therapies, etc.).

Results achieved with internal quality management measures (indicator monitoring; establishment of quality circles or committees including, e.g., mortality conferences analyzing quality issues; and discussing, implementing, and monitoring the implementation of corrective measures) shall be documented in annual quality reports to be established by all public and private facilities offering secondary level care (again, the availability of such reports could become a licensing or accreditation criterion).

With regard to external quality management, the DOH (quality department) shall collect data from all hospitals on selected indicators and analyze those data by comparing the results achieved by the hospitals and their core services against each other. Of course, this process will need to take into consideration the patient mix the hospitals are dealing with to avoid bias in the evaluation due to "cream skimming" by health care providers (e.g., through early transfer to tertiary level hospitals) and other measures to purposely or unintentionally manipulate data on clinical outcomes. Such kind of benchmarking will help both health care facility managers and the DOH to monitor and improve the quality of care.

Continuous Medical Education

Last but not least, the protocols and pathways and systematic quality management processes and related tools and instrument at health care facilities require regular updating of knowledge and skills of all medical, paramedical, technical, and administrative staff through training and other capacity-building measures (e.g., e-learning courses; on-site supervision, coaching, or mentoring; peer review of medical records and clinical practice; staff exchange programs; and certified training offered by national and international third-party providers).

Participation in such measures and events should be mandatory to all staff and be documented or monitored through a credit points account. Training and other capacity-building measures, if officially recognized, are being scored through a credit point system. Each staff is required to get a minimum number of credit points during 24 months to maintain their license as a medical or paramedical professional; for other staff, incentives could be given to those who achieve the required minimum number of credit points.

The purpose of this approach is to make people understand that for quality care, continuous professional and human resources development is indispensable and that this is everybody's responsibility (provided that employers and public authorities will offer the opportunity to participate in or organize related measures and events). This approach would include financial support to participation as required and appropriate. Continuous medical education has to get its budget line from the hospital budget plans.

Box A1: World Health Organization Health Systems Framework and Quality of Care

The role of leadership and governance for health care quality, both at policy and operational levels, is indispensable. A strategically developed health care financing system needs to link the financing of public health care services with their quality (in terms of process quality and impact on the individual's and the population's health status). One of the results-oriented models of health care financing was the Rahim Yar Khan District (Punjab Province) model introduced in 2003, where the responsibility for providing primary health care (PHC) services was handed over to the Punjab Rural Support Program, a nongovernment organization (NGO) that was contracted to overcome the underutilization of services and the absenteeism of doctors assigned in basic health units (BHUs) and rural health centers (RHCs). Despite controversial viewpoints and discussions around this model, the outcomes of the project showed higher utilization rates together with improved physical conditions of BHUs and lower levels of out-of-pocket spending among the community. However, the quality of services observed during the external evaluation of the program[a] indicated the need to define a minimum package of PHC services and standards that have to be included in the contractual arrangement with the service provider and the need to strengthen capacities for monitoring and evaluating provider performance and service quality needs with the Department of Health (DOH) before moving to further roll out such initiatives.

A similar results-oriented approach to health care financing but for hospital services has been introduced in Khyber Pakhtunkhwa with the KfW Development Bank-supported social health insurance initiative.[b] Hospitals receive a diagnosis-related group like lump sum for inpatient treatment. However, the financing scheme is facing similar weaknesses, impacting on the quality of care: the amount paid is being negotiated between the hospital (the service provider) and the organization managing the social health insurance scheme (the purchaser of health services), and there are significant differences in the amount that is being paid for the same diagnosis and there is a lack of standards defining how and what kind of services are to be provided under a specific diagnosis (leading to a "buying a pig in a poke" effect).

Quality of care is closely interlinked with human resources performance and thus with health workforce issues in general. After years of emphasis on training doctors, the overall availability of medical doctors corresponds with the World Health Organization (WHO) minimum requirement of 1 doctor per 1,000 population, but with significant discrepancies between urban (1.45/1,000) and rural (0.36/1,000) areas (data from the WHO Global Atlas of the Health Workforce 2015) and a continuing lack of specialists, including in areas such as health care management and public health. The nurse-to-doctor ratio is still far below the WHO recommended ratio of 4:1 (0.38 per 1,000 population, with 0.76 in urban and 0.29 in rural areas) indicating the gap and neglect of paramedical training, which needs to be reinforced. As mentioned above, various strategies are being experimented in different provinces of Pakistan to improve performance and quality of services provided by medical and paramedical staff at public facilities, including outsourcing and public–private redeployment; merit-based recruitment and retention mechanisms; and autonomy in human resources management, which has been granted to health care facilities in Khyber Pakhtunkhwa since 2002.

continued on next page

Box A1 *continued*

Considering the rather rapid changes in medical knowledge and technology and related diagnostic and therapeutic procedures, continuous professional and medical education to maintain and further develop competencies and skills is specifically relevant for health care quality. Continuous education is not yet systematically introduced in Pakistan's health system—an issue that will have to be addressed in a human resources for health (HRH) policy that needs to be part of and support any strategy aiming at improved quality of care. Such a policy may also include a licensing system with informal or nonqualified health care providers ("traditional healers") who will have to be trained in the screening for and recognition of serious health problems that would require modern medical care to save the patient's life and/or to avoid grave damage to the patient's physical and/or mental well-being.

Various forms of malpractice in the chain of production, supply, and prescription of drugs and other medical products, including inappropriate registration, collusion of interest in pricing, lack or overlooking of (quality) control mechanisms and procedures, and the attitude of many doctors to establish multi-pragmatic drug treatment schemes have serious impact on the quality of care both in terms of efficacy of the prescribed treatment and efficiency (nonrational use of limited resources, mainly out-of-pocket spending, thus affecting especially the poor). The regulatory framework needs to be revised, updated, and enforced to protect the population's health and secure rational use of funds (which is a major criterion for the quality of a public health care system).

Budget constraints have led to slow adoption of medical technologies, specifically in secondary care level public health facilities. This constraint is relevant for diagnostic procedures (laboratory, imaging), for which patients have to use private sector facilities, which further aggravates the inequalities in access to quality care. It is also important that health and hospital information systems including tools like electronic patient record (EPR) (i) help continuously monitor and evaluate inputs and outcomes of medical care (both in clinical and economic terms, thus promoting research in health technology assessment); and (ii) provide an excellent instrument to improve quality of care through standardization of diagnostic and therapeutic procedures (using predefined clinical pathways) and through computer-assisted drug prescription to avoid undesired side effects due to wrong dosage or combination of drugs or mixing up of patients, which together are the most frequent forms of medical errors and causes of premature (in-hospital) deaths.[c]

Apart from utilization data, there is little information available based on routine data to assess the quality of service delivery—not in the public sector and certainly not in the private sector. Various forms of malpractice, staff absenteeism and dual (public–private) job holding, unauthorized payments requested from patients, and generally the low level of quality due to limited resources for investments in improved infrastructure, equipment, and qualification of human resources characterize the situation in the health sector in general and in the hospital sector in particular.

---

[a]   B. Loevinsohn. 2006. Partnering with NGOs to Strengthen Management: An External Evaluation of the Chief Minister's Initiative on Primary Health Care in Rahim Yar Khan District, Punjab. *South Asia Human Development Sector Series*. No. 13. Washington, DC: World Bank.

[b]   Financial Cooperation between the Federal Republic of Germany and the Islamic Republic of Pakistan; BMZ no. 2013 66 228: Preparatory Study for the Social Health Protection Project Phase II; Final Report, management4health, Frankfurt am Main, September 2017.

[c]   Institute of Medicine. 2000. *To Err is Human: Building a Safer Health System*. Washington, DC: The National Academies Press.

Appendix 5—Financing Sources by Financing Agents, FY2016

PRs million

Financing Agents			Financing Sources								Total	%
			Public Funds				Private Funds			Official Donor Agencies		
			Government Funds			Autonomous Bodies	Employer Funds	Household Funds	Local NGO			
			Federal Government	Provincial Government	District/Tehsil Bodies							
General Government	Federal government	Federal government (civil)										
		Military health expenditures	3,186								3,186	2.73
	Provincial government	Department	Health		15,416							15,416	13.22
		Other		209							209	0.18
		Population Welfare		20							20	0.02
	District bodies	District government									0	0.00
		Cantonment boards			120						120	0.10
	Social security funds through government	ESSI[a]					345				345	0.30
		Zakat health expenditures						109			109	0.09
Territorial government	Bait-ul-Mal						63			63	0.05
Autonomous bodies and corporations						146					146	0.13

continued on next page

Table *continued*

Financing Agents	Public Funds				Private Funds			Official Donor Agencies	Total	%
	Government Funds		District/Tehsil Bodies	Autonomous Bodies	Employer Funds	Household Funds	Local NGO			
	Federal Government	Provincial Government								
	PRs million									
Private Sector Private households' out-of-pocket payment						84,232			84,232	72.26
Local nongovernment organizations (NGOs)							11,702		11,702	10.04
Official donor agencies								1,020	1,020	0.88
Total	**3,186**	**15,645**	**120**	**146**	**345**	**84,404**	**11,702**	**1,020**	**116,568**	**100.00**
%	2.73	13.42	0.10	0.13	0.30	72.41	10.04	0.88	100.00[b]	

ESSI = Employees Social Security Institution.

Notes:

[a] Social security funds from employers.

[b] Percentage may not total 100% because of rounding.

Source: Estimations by Chief Statistical Officer Ihsan ul Haq, National Health Accounts, Pakistan Bureau of Statistics.

Appendix 6—Overview of Population Segments Receiving Financial Coverage for Health

| | **Formally Employed Sector** | | | | | | | |
	Federal Government	**Provincial Government**	**Military**	**Cantonment Boards**	**Autonomous Bodies (Federal and Provincial)**	**Private Health Insurance**	**Employees Social Security Institution**	**Total**
Sources of finance	General taxation	General taxation	General taxation	General taxation	General taxation plus profits raised by the organizations	Voluntary contributions (premiums) paid by individuals and employers for the group insurance of their employees	Employer's contribution (7% of employee's salary) toward health insurance of employees	
Population covered	Federal government provides health coverage to its employees and their dependents.	Provincial government provides health coverage to its employees and their dependents.	Military provides health coverage to its employees and their dependents.	Cantonment boards provide health coverage to its employees and their dependents.	Autonomous bodies provide health coverage to its employees and their dependents.	Individuals and employers voluntarily opt for health insurance of their employees.	Under an ordinance, it's compulsory for all the establishments that employ 10 or more persons to provide health insurance to their employees and their dependents.	
Total number of beneficiaries / employees and their dependents (in millions)	0.99[a]	3.05[b]	2.04[c]	0.23[d]	0.85[e]	0.10[f]	0.58[g]	7.84

continued on next page

Table continued

	Formally Employed Sector							
	Federal Government	Provincial Government	Military	Cantonment Boards	Autonomous Bodies (Federal and Provincial)	Private Health Insurance	Employees Social Security Institution	Total
Services covered	Both outpatient and inpatient, but there is no explicit package for inpatient services	Both outpatient and inpatient, but there is no explicit package for inpatient services	Both outpatient and inpatient, but there is no explicit package for inpatient services	Both outpatient and inpatient, but there is no explicit package for inpatient services	Both outpatient and inpatient, but there is no explicit package for inpatient services	Usually, no outpatient service is covered. There is a financial cap on the covered inpatient services.	Both outpatient and inpatient services, and there is a financial cap on the latter	
Single or multiple purchasers	Single purchaser	Single purchaser	Single purchaser	Single purchaser	Single purchaser	Multiple purchasers	Single purchaser	
Types of providers from whom services are purchased	Mostly public. In case of nonavailability of services in the public sector, services are approved from the private sector on a case-by-case basis.	Mostly public. In case of nonavailability of services in the public sector, services are approved from the private sector on a case-by-case basis.	All the staff and their dependents are entitled to get both outpatient and inpatient services from military hospitals (including secondary and tertiary hospitals).	Primary health care centers and military hospitals in respective cantonments	Hospitals owned and run by autonomous agencies and public hospitals. Services can be availed of from private hospitals on a case-by-case basis.	Private hospitals	Dispensaries, hospitals, and treatment centers owned and run by ESSI	
Provider payment mechanism	Fee for service	Fee for service	Fee for service	Fee for service		Payments against agreed treatment packages	Fee for service	

continued on next page

Table continued

	Informally Employed Sector				
	Sehat Sahulat Program	**Bait-ul-Mal**	**Zakat**	**Others (NGOs, Foundations)**	**Total**
Sources of finance	General taxation	General taxation	Muslims' social security fund generated through 2.5% deductions on annual bank account savings	Individual philanthropy plus local and foreign donations	
Population covered	Households below poverty line of $2, persons with disabilities, and transgenders	A social safety net for providing individual assistance to widows, destitute women, orphans, the disabled, and the poor not covered through Zakat	A social safety net for providing individual assistance to widows, destitute women, orphans, the disabled, and the poor	Mostly for vulnerable populations (migrants, those prone to earthquakes and floods, etc.)	
Total number of beneficiaries / employees and their dependents covered (in millions)	19.20[h]	0.0023[i]	0.030[j]	0.09[k]	19.32
Services covered	Inpatient (all illnesses requiring hospitalization in secondary hospitals, and selected treatments in tertiary hospitals)	Mostly inpatient (illnesses requiring hospitalization in secondary and tertiary hospitals) and high-cost diagnostics	Mostly illnesses requiring admissions in secondary hospitals and low-cost diagnostics	A broad variation in the set of services supported by different organizations	
Single or multiple purchasers	Single purchaser	Single purchaser	Single purchaser	Multiple purchasers	

continued on next page

Table continued

| | Informally Employed Sector | | | | |
	Sehat Sahulat Program	Bait-ul-Mal	Zakat	Others (NGOs, Foundations)	Total
Types of providers from whom services are purchased	Both public and private hospitals	Only public. In case of nonavailability of services in the public sector, services are approved from the private sector on a case-by-case basis	Only public. In case of nonavailability of services in the public sector, services are approved from the private sector on a case-by-case basis	Both public and private hospitals	
Provider payment mechanism	Payment against agreed treatment packages plus fee for additional services	Fee for service	Fee for service	Fee for service	

ESSI = Employees Social Security Institution, NGO = nongovernment organization.

Notes:

[a] Total number of federal government employees in Khyber Pakhtunkhwa was obtained from the *Annual Statistical Bulletin of Federal Government Employees 2012–13* and multiplied by the average household size (7.9) in the province.

[b] Total number of employees of the Government of Khyber Pakhtunkhwa was obtained from the Department of Finance and multiplied by the average household size (7.9) in the province.

[c] Total number of armed forces employees and their dependents in 2009–2010 was obtained from the medical directorate, general headquarters, Rawalpindi. This figure has been raised by population growth (2.4%) to get the estimated number of employees and their dependents for 2017–2018. Based on the % of total employees of other federal organizations residing in Khyber Pakhtunkhwa and security situation in the province, it has been assumed that 28% of the total armed forces employees and their dependents are residing in Khyber Pakhtunkhwa.

[d] The other NGO is likely an underreported figure, as it only includes patients treated in Peshawar cantonment hospitals. Source: Cantonment Board Peshawar. http://www.cbp.gov.pk.

[e] The total number of employees in autonomous bodies was obtained from establishment division publication 2012–2013. About 15.18% of the total employees were in Khyber Pakhtunkhwa. This number was multiplied by the average household size (7.9) in the province.

[f] Estimates were obtained from the data shared by private health insurance companies (Source: The Insurance Association of Pakistan).

[g] Khyber Pakhtunkhwa Employees Social Security Institution.

[h] Khyber Pakhtunkhwa Sehat Sahulat Program.

[i] Pakistan Bait-ul-Mal.

[j] Zakat & Ushr Department, Government of Khyber Pakhtunkhwa.

[k] Estimations were made based on Pakistan Centre for Philanthropy data.

Source: Estimations by Chief Statistical Officer Ihsan ul Haq, National Health Accounts, Pakistan Bureau of Statistics.

Appendix 7—Social Health Protection Initiative: Sehat Sahulat Program

a) Goal and Objectives

The overall goal of the program is to improve the health status of the targeted population through increased access to quality health services and to reduce poverty through reduced out-of-pocket (OOP) payments for health expenditures.

b) Program Targets

The social health protection initiative (SHPI) has the following targets:

1. About 69% of the population in the province have free health insurance.
2. OOP expenditure of the enrolled population for inpatient care is reduced by at least 50%.
3. The utilization rate of hospital care has increased by 3%–4% in the insured population.

Identification and Targeting of Beneficiaries

Proxy means testing (PMT), the targeting mechanism developed by Benazir Income Support Programme, is being used to identify beneficiary households, which are exempted from paying health insurance premiums.[7] Households whose PMT score is 32.49 or below are eligible to be enrolled.

Each registered household is given a health card (Sehat Insaf card), which makes them eligible for availing benefits of the program. Each household can enroll up to eight members. The head of the household, spouse, and children are enrolled as priority, followed by dependent parents living in the same house. However, as noted in the Department of Health (DOH) *Year Book 2016-17*, the average household size in Khyber Pakhtunkhwa is 7.9.

Premium and Benefits

Premium is PRs1,499 ($12.96) per household per year and is being paid by the Government of Khyber Pakhtunkhwa to State Life Insurance Corporation of Pakistan (SLIC). In case of unutilized premium, 80% has to be returned to provincial government at the end of the year, while SLIC can retain 20% as profit. Each registered household is getting coverage up to PRs240,000 ($2,076) per household (PRs30,000 or $259 per person) per annum for secondary care for all the illnesses requiring hospitalization at district-level hospitals, and up to PRs300,000 ($2,594) per household for tertiary care. Pre- and post-hospitalization care up to 1 day before hospitalization and up to 5 days from the date of discharge from the hospital is also part of the package. Tertiary care diseases include

(i)   heart and vascular diseases;
(ii) complications of diabetes mellitus requiring hospitalization;

---

[7] World Bank. Measuring Income and Poverty Using Proxy Means Tests. https://olc.worldbank.org/sites/default/files/1.pdf. "Proxy Means Test allows us to estimate the income or consumption when precise measurements are unavailable or difficult to obtain. In many situations, we might not be able to tell how much a family earns or spends every month. Even the household members themselves might not be able to tell— they seldom maintain detailed records." An example of a proxy would be ownership of a motorcycle, which reflects that a certain level of income is coming into the household that not only allows for the purchase of the motorcycle but also for its maintenance and usage. In the case of Benazir Income Support Programme, a poverty scorecard, which contained various proxies, was used to assess the poverty level of the household, and, based on this card, a score was assigned to each household. Any family at or below the threshold of 32.49 was included in the SHPI.

(iii) emergency and trauma including all types of fractures, head injuries, and spinal injuries;
(iv) all types of cancers;
(v) hepatitis B and hepatitis C complications; and
(vi) organ failure management including kidney transplants.

Additional benefits include

(i) wage replacement of PRs250 ($2.16) per day for a maximum of 3 days to be paid upon discharge;
(ii) transportation costs for seeking tertiary care of PRs2,000 ($17.30) to be paid upon discharge;
(iii) transportation costs for seeking maternity care of PRs1,000 ($8.65) to be paid upon discharge (in case of normal or surgical delivery);
(iv) one outpatient department (OPD) voucher to each beneficiary upon discharge, which can be utilized for one post-discharge follow-up visit; and
(v) burial insurance of PRs10,000 ($86.48) in case of the death of a beneficiary during admission.

To cover costs exceeding the specified limit, the government has created a reserve fund of PRs120 million ($1.04 million) through the payment of PRs50 ($0.43) per household per year to SLIC. Table below shows the overview of phases of the social protection initiative.

Table A2: Overview of Phases of the Social Health Protection Initiative (Sehat Sahulat Program)

Salient Features	SSP (Phase I)	SSP (Phase II)	SSP (Phase 2 with extension) / Phase III
Area	Four districts	Entire province	Entire province
Total funding	PRs1.4 billion ($12.1 million)	PRs5.4 billion ($46.7 million)	PRs6.5 billion ($56.2 million) Additional cost of PRs1.1 billion ($9.5 million)
Source of funding	KfW + Government of Khyber Pakhtunkhwa	Government of Khyber Pakhtunkhwa	Government of Khyber Pakhtunkhwa
Funding	Total cost: PRs1.4 billion KfW share: PRs1,233.2 million (88%) Government share: PRs165.9 million (12%)	Total cost around PRs5.4 billion, all through government's general revenue	Total cost around PRs5.4 billion, all through government's general revenue
Who Is Covered?			
Percentage of population	21% poorest population of target districts	51% poorest population of entire province	69% poorest population of entire province
Enrollment criterion	Families with PMT score of 16.7 or less	Families with PMT score of 24.5 or less	Families with PMT score of 32.5 or less
Family size	7 persons per household	8 persons per household	8 persons per household
Total population covered	0.7 million (0.1 million households with 7 members each)	14.4 million (1.8 million households with 8 members each)	19.2 million (2.4 million households with 8 members each)
What Is Covered?			
Type of services	Inpatient services only	Predominantly inpatient services	Predominantly inpatient services
Outpatient cover	Maternity services only	Maternity services and cancer care	Maternity services and cancer care
Secondary diseases	Almost all are covered, needing admission	All secondary health conditions needing admission	All secondary health conditions needing admission
Tertiary conditions	None	Yes, limited tertiary cover	Yes, limited tertiary cover

PMT = proxy means testing, SSP = Sehat Sahulat Program.

Source: Sheraz Ahmad, Social Health Protection Initiative (SHPI). Personal communication, January 2018.

Appendix 8—Actuarial Projections of Supply and Demand-Side Interventions in the Khyber Pakhtunkhwa Health Sector

In FY2018, the total allocation for the health sector is PRs66.47 billion ($574.83 million), an increase of 22% compared with the previous year, and accounts for 11.02% of the total budget of the Government of Khyber Pakhtunkhwa, a small 0.4% increase compared with the previous year.

In 2015, the provincial government launched the social health protection initiative (SHPI) as a micro health insurance in four districts with the financial support of the German government through KfW. The establishment of the SHPI, expansion into all districts, and enlargement of the percentage of the population covered by SHPI were significant steps toward achieving universal health coverage (UHC). As of FY2018, the premium for up to 69% of the population (i.e., the poor) is to be paid by the provincial government for inpatient secondary and tertiary health care services.

While the SHPI is successful in bringing access to inpatient health care to a large percentage of the province's population, at the end of 2017 not all of the nominally eligible 69% of the population had been enrolled. Furthermore, the empaneled public and private health facilities where members can access their SHPI-provided health care only represent about 53% of all hospitals providing inpatient services.[8]

Next to the SHPI, there are some initiatives including private health insurances in Khyber Pakhtunkhwa. Assuming that all stated coverages are realized and that there is no overlap between population segments, then about 95% of the population are entitled to some form of health insurance.

In an actuarial model, the total health costs of the entire province are estimated at PRs173.1 billion ($1.5 billion) in FY2018 and are projected to increase to PRs1,209.4 billion ($10.5 billion) by FY2036. The largest share consists of the costs for human resources for health (HRH). In terms of levels of health care and outpatient versus inpatient services, the costs for primary health care (outpatient) increase the fastest, from PRs38.8 billion ($335.5 million) in FY2018 to a projected PRs396.9 billion ($3.4 billion) in FY2036.

However, the budget of the Department of Health (DOH) that is available[9] for health care provision is projected to increase from PRs51.7 billion ($447.1 million) in the FY2018 to PRs111.2 billion ($961.7 million) in FY2036. The DOH budget for health care provision is insufficient to pay for all services (outpatient, inpatient, from primary to tertiary care, and in public and private sectors). Another interpretation of this result is that the DOH budget is insufficient to provide a complete UHC.

Moreover, when considering a limited UHC for 69% of the population—covering the costs for the provision of primary health care (PHC) outpatient care, secondary outpatient and inpatient

---

[8] F. Ng. 2018. *Khyber Pakhtunkhwa Planning for Physical and Human Resources*. Background paper for the Assessment of the Khyber Pakhtunkhwa Health Sector. Peshawar. 13–15 February.

[9] This is the DOH annual budget after subtracting grants and transfers as well as the overhead for administrative staff and public health, as such it might be interpreted as an upper limit to the available budget for health services provision within the DOH budget.

services, and a limited scope of tertiary outpatient and inpatient services at public and private health care providers—there is a deficit in FY2018 of PRs24.4 billion ($211.0 million), which is projected to reach PRs482.3 billion ($4.2 billion) in FY2036. In other words, the DOH's budget is insufficient to provide even a "limited UHC" benefits package to the poor.

The estimated cost of the SHPI of PRs24.0 billion ($207.6 million) in FY2018 is more than three times higher than the budget for Phase II of the SHPI of PRs6.5 billion ($56.2 million). Should the aim of the premium of the SHPI be to cover the full costs of the SHPI program (assuming all eligible people are enrolled and have meaningful access to health care), then the premium would need to quadruple in FY2018 to PRs6,177 ($53.42) per household per annum, which is projected to increase to PRs27,108 ($234.43) in FY2036.

The current health infrastructure of Khyber Pakhtunkhwa is inadequate (footnote 8) to deliver the health services needed by the population. In terms of infrastructure (buildings, equipment), there is a clear lack of health care especially at the referral levels—the secondary and tertiary health care levels. Assuming that all required health care infrastructure to develop the province's health sector into a sector at par with developed health infrastructure sectors of industrialized countries can be built and equipped within a year and excluding HRH costs, then a gap of PRs433.7 billion ($3.8 billion) in funding appears. What this hypothetical exercise shows is the need to invest in the health care infrastructure to assure continuous supply-side readiness, especially once the enrolled members start consuming their benefits under SHPI.